THE BETHLEM & MAUDSLEY NHS TRUST

PRESCRIBING GUIDELINES

GU00806290

The Maudsley

Advancing Mental Health Care

THE BETHLEM & MAUDSLEY NHS TRUST

PRESCRIBING GUIDELINES

5th Edition

1999

MARTIN DUNITZ

© Taylor, McConnell, McConnell, Abel, Kerwin 1999

First published in the United Kingdom in 1999 by

Martin Dunitz Ltd
The Livery House
7–9 Pratt Street
London NW1 0AE

A CIP record for this book is available from the British Library.

ISBN 1–85317–835–7

Printed and bound in Great Britain by the University Press, Cambridge, UK.

Authors and Contributors

David Taylor – Senior Editor / Author
Chief Pharmacist, Bethlem and Maudsley NHS Trust
Honorary Senior Lecturer, Institute of Psychiatry

Denise McConnell (née Duncan) – Managing Editor / Author
Senior Drug Information Pharmacist
Bethlem and Maudsley NHS Trust

Harry McConnell – Editor / Author
Psychiatrist/Neurologist
Chairman, TEAM (*T*owards *E*ducation for *A*ll with *M*ultimedia) /
EEI (*E*pilepsy *E*ducational *I*nitiative)
Research Fellow, Institute of Psychiatry

Kathryn Abel – Author
MRC Research Fellow, Honorary Senior Registrar
Bethlem and Maudsley NHS Trust

Founding Editor:
Robert Kerwin
Professor of Clinical Neuropharmacology, Institute of Psychiatry
Consultant Psychiatrist, Bethlem and Maudsley NHS Trust

Graphics and Text Design: As'ad Abu Khalil, TEAM

Disclaimer

The opinions expressed are those of the individual authors in consultation with various international experts and with the Bethlem and Maudsley NHS Trust's Drug and Therapeutics Committee. Every care has been taken to assure that these Guidelines are up-to-date and accurate. However, it must be considered that this document is but the end product of reasoned influences from several clinicians. We do not claim that every piece of advice provided is "correct", only that we have taken care to ensure that advice is based on firm evidence and clinical experience. We hope to have included all information available to us in January 1999, but this will inevitably become outdated as time goes by. Readers should bear this in mind and should always consult the latest manufacturers' information and the British National Formulary or the equivalent text for their country of practice.

It is also important to recognise that Clinical Practice differs from one country to another and that availability and licensing of drugs discussed in these Guidelines also vary with geographical location. Please note that many of the drugs listed in the tables are done so alphabetically and not necessarily in order of preference. Generic drugs may require special care and attention in relation to dosage and use. Special attention should always be paid to contraindications and side effects. Many of the drugs discussed are not yet available in some countries and many of the uses may be "off licence" in the UK as well as overseas. Clinicians are strongly advised to check their local laws and local hospital or national clinical guidelines before using any information in a clinical situation. The clinical care of any individual patient remains at all times that of the treating psychiatrist or other clinician. Additional terms and conditions may apply and may be notified. All regulatory bodies will be those of the United Kingdom and the law of England will apply in all matters relating to the Maudsley Prescribing Guidelines. No liability is accepted for any injury, loss or damage howsoever caused.

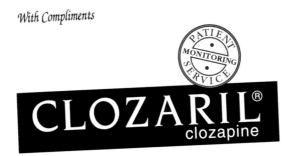

With Compliments

Contents:

III. Treatment of Affective Illness

IV. Treatment of Anxiety

V. Treatment of Special Patient Populations

VII. Adverse Effects of Psychotropic Drugs

Preface

The Maudsley Prescribing Guidelines have now been produced for five years, having begun as a ten-page pamphlet designed to be of use to prescribers in our Trust. This 5th edition of the Guidelines is the first to be formally published and distributed by a bona fide publisher. It has been fully updated and expanded to meet, it is hoped, the needs of prescribers, nursing staff, pharmacists and other professions allied to medicine.

The Guidelines are written and refined by the authors and founding editor over a period of twelve to eighteen months. The finished product, however, is the result of a great many influences drawn from a number of clinicians with a variety of experiences and specialist knowledge. Without the input of these people, *The Guidelines* would be palpably impoverished. We are therefore greatly indebted to all those who contributed to former editions and to Professors Stuart Checkley, Channi Kumar, Eric Taylor, Chris Cook, Trevor Silverstone, Ed Coffey, Sigurd Ackerman, Sarah Romans and Peter J. Snyder as well as Drs. Rod Pipe, Eric Fombonne, Simon Fleminger, Kapil Sayal, Mike Farrell, Simon Lovestone, Marika Bogyi, Ibrahim Al-Khodair, Pat McElhatton, Ken Barrett and Janet Treasure and Jat Harchowal, Kate Trotter, Lucy Reeves, Fiona Woods, Ann Hutton and Eromona Whiskey who have helped substantially with this 5th edition. The antipsychotic prescribing guidelines were largely developed by senior clinicians of the Bethlem and Maudsley Trust and approved by the Trust's Medical Committee.

In developing the Guidelines over the years, two important observations have frequently been made. First, it is clear that there are few unarguable "correct answers" in psychopharmacology. What we present here is the end product of reasoned influences from several clinicians: it is simply well-considered opinion. We do not claim that every piece of advice provided is "correct", only that we have taken care to ensure that advice is based on firm evidence and clinical experience. Second, things change. In fact, in psychopharmacology, things change very quickly. We hope to have included all information available to us in January 1999, but this will inevitably become outdated as time goes by. Readers should bear this in mind and should always consult the latest manufacturers' information and the British National Formulary. Remember also that where drugs are used outside their product licence, the prescriber bears legal responsibility.

David Taylor
January 1999

I

Principles of

Psychotropic Prescribing

3
General Principles

◆   The decision to use drug therapy must take into account the potential risks and benefits of treatment to the patient. These should be discussed with the patient and/or their carer along with treatment options.

◆   A full evaluation of the patient's symptoms should be undertaken by the clinician before prescribing, including mental status and physical examination and laboratory tests. It is important to clarify the diagnosis since many illnesses may present as depression, psychosis or anxiety.

◆   Use of drug combinations (polypharmacy) should be avoided whenever possible. When combination therapy is necessary, attention should be given to both pharmacodynamic and pharmacokinetic interactions and drug choices made accordingly.

◆   In general, the lowest effective dose of a drug should be used.

◆   Titration of most psychotropic agents should be done gradually and weaning of them should also be done slowly in chronic and subacute conditions. In acute situations, choice of drug will depend in part on how rapidly it may be titrated for a given clinical situation. The rate of titration and of weaning will vary depending on the class of drug and how long a patient has been taking the drug. One should be aware of those psychotropics which may cause a discontinuation syndrome or which may cause rebound symptoms or withdrawal phenomena.

◆   In switching from one psychotropic to another the clinician must take into account the half-life of the drug being discontinued, the potential for discontinuation symptoms and any potential interactions (pharmacokinetic and pharmacodynamic) with the new agent.

◆   In discontinuing psychotropics in patients one must consider the length of time a patient has been on the drug as well as the issues of physical and psychological withdrawal. For some drugs (e.g.. antiepileptic drugs, benzodiazepines) it may be appropriate to withdraw agents over many months. Others may be discontinued abruptly or withdrawn over days / weeks.

Use of Laboratory Monitoring

The history, mental status examination and physical examination form the cornerstone of psychiatric diagnosis and are key to monitoring of prescribing and following a patient's progress. It is often necessary, however, to use a variety of laboratory tests, EEG and neuroimaging to assist in the diagnosis and treatment of psychiatric illness. The following table outlines some of the more helpful blood tests and their relevance to psychiatric practice.

Laboratory Tests and their Relevance in Psychiatry

(modified from McConnell 1998)

Test	Comments
WBC count and differential	Important for evaluating the possibility of: (1) infectious diseases, (2) leukaemia, and (3) leucopenia due to certain psychotropic medications. This is particularly important for the monitoring of clozapine therapy (see below)
RBC count, Hemoglobin, Hematocrit	Important for evaluating polycythemia and anaemia, which may relate to a variety of psychotropics
Mean corpuscular volume (MCV)	Is the average volume of a RBC; useful in establishing whether an anaemia is macrocytic (ie, increased, such as in alcoholism, folate and B12 deficiency – often related to AEDs) or microcytic (i.e. decreased, such as in iron deficiency anaemia – sometimes related to NSAIDs)
Reticulocyte count	Gives an indication of RBC production and, hence, of bone marrow activity; increased in anaemias secondary to blood loss or hemolysis, decreased in anaemias secondary to impairment of RBC maturation (e.g. folate, B12 related to AEDs; iron deficiency anaemias before treatment)
Platelets	May be decreased due to drugs (e.g. valproate, phenothiazines) or due to medical illness; may occur along with other cell lines (pancytopenia)
Erythrocyte sedimentation rate (ESR)	A non-specific index of inflammation; elevated in infectious, neoplastic and inflammatory (e.g. vasculitis, systemic lupus erythematosus) illness
Coagulation tests	May be elevated in liver disease of many causes; Prothrombin time (PT), International normalized ratio (INR) used to monitor warfarin therapy; partial thromboplastin time (PTT) and activated partial thromboplastin time (APTT) used to monitor heparin therapy; need to be monitored closely in patients on warfarin taking psychotropics because of interactions (see section V)

RBC and serum folate; Vitamin B12 levels	Serum levels of folate and B12 used to screen for deficiency of these important vitamins; deficiency may present with or without concomitant anaemia with a variety of mental state changes (depression, psychosis, cognitive deficits, dementia) and/or neurological sequelae; deficiency may occur due to impaired absorption, deficient intake or secondary to medication (e.g. antiepileptic drugs); RBC folate should be monitored as it is more indicative of overall status than serum levels. The Schillings test and serum intrinsic factor are useful in evaluating B12 deficiency due to pernicious anaemia; it is important to monitor both B12 and folate as treatment with folate alone may reverse haematological abnormalities (macrocytic anaemia) without reversal of neurological deficits. Neurological and psychiatric manifestations of folate and B12 deficiency can occur with a normal haematological profile. Folate and B12 are affected by many drugs, particularly AEDs including phenytoin, carbamazepine and valproate. They should be measured in patients on these drugs as they are common contributors to psychiatric comorbidity and need to be supplemented appropriately. This is particularly important in women of child-bearing age where folate should be considered before conception (see section V for discussion of folate supplementation)
Thyroid Function Tests	Thyroid-stimulating hormone (TSH) is best screening test; serum triiodothyronine (T3), thyroxine (T4), reverse T3, T3 resin uptake (T3RU), free T4, free thyroxine index (FTI), antithyroglobulin antibodies and microsomal antibodies are also useful in the further evaluation of thyroid illness. Thyroid testing should be done to evaluate possible medication-induced thyroid disease (e.g. carbamazepine, lithium). Hypo- and hyper-thyroidism can present with a variety of psychiatric presentations, with improvement in mental state changes often lagging behind improvement in biochemical parameters
Dexamethasone Suppression Test (DST)	Measurement of serum cortisol checked at specific times before and after the administration of 1 mg dexamethasone, thought by some to be a biological marker for depression; a normal response, however, does not rule out the possibility of depression and an abnormal response must similarly be interpreted in the clinical context; may be useful in some ambiguous situations
Prolactin	Useful in evaluating patients on antipsychotics with galactorrhoea or to evaluate compliance, as antipsychotics characteristically increase prolactin; management of hyperprolactinaemia due to psychotropics is discussed in section VII; may be of limited use in evaluating nonepileptic seizure-like events (NESLEs) if psychotropics are controlled for and if sample is obtained within 20 minutes of a suspected seizure – a normal value, however, should not be interpreted as representing a NESLE, as no rise in levels may occur in seizures related to epilepsy as well. A clear rise in baseline within 20 min. of a seizure is useful as an indication of the seizure relating to epilepsy

Laboratory Tests and their Relevance in Psychiatry *(Continued)*

Electrolytes	Sodium (Na⁺), potassium (K⁺), chloride (Cl⁻), and bicarbonate (HCO₃⁻) are all useful screening tests in psychiatric illness and should also be monitored in patients on psychotropics (esp. carbamazepine and antidepressants) which may cause hyponatraemia; hyponatraemia is also seen in various medical illnesses and in SIADH and psychogenic polydipsia; hypokalaemia is common in people with bulimia and anorexia
Liver Function Tests	Useful screening test in psychiatric patients and also to be monitored in patients on psychotropics which may affect liver function (esp. antiepileptic drugs); includes alanine aminotransferase (ALT), alkaline phosphatase (AP), aspartate aminotransferase (AST), gamma-glutamyl transaminase (GGT) and lactate dehydrogenase (LDH) which has five isoenzymes and may be elevated in other medical conditions as well; GGT most sensitive of these; bilirubin (total, direct and indirect) useful in evaluation of hepatobiliary disease and haemolytic anaemia and may have to be ordered separately in some labs
Renal Function Tests	Blood urea nitrogen (BUN) and creatinine both elevated in renal failure; should be monitored in patients on lithium and amantadine
Amylase and lipase levels	Used to evaluate pancreatitis and pancreatic carcinoma; should be screened in patients on valproate with any gastrointestinal symptoms as this may induce pancreatitis; may also be a useful measure in monitoring bulimia
Glucose	Important test in evaluating both the possibility of diabetes mellitus as well as hypoglycaemia, which may present with a variety of intermittent mental state changes, including delirium and psychosis
Creatinine phosphokinase (CPK)	Useful in evaluating possible neuroleptic malignant syndrome (NMS) – see section VII for discussion.
Copper and ceruloplasmin	Used to diagnose and evaluate Wilson's disease which is an inherited alteration in copper metabolism which presents with personality changes, altered cognition affective symptoms or psychosis associated with a movement disorder, usually in adolescents and young adults

Porphyrins	Porphobilinogen (PBG) aminolevulinic acid (ALA) and other porphyrins and metabolites used to diagnose porphyria, an inherited metabolic disorder which can present with intermittent psychosis and/or seizures or other neuropsychiatric manifestations; important as many psychotropics will exacerbate porphyria (see section V)
LE prep	Used along with other tests, including antinuclear antibodies (ANA), anti-DNA antibodies, lupus anticoagulant, and complement levels in the diagnosis of systemic lupus erythematosus (SLE); may present with depression, delirium, psychosis or dementia; phenothiazines, amongst other drugs, may cause false positives
RBC transketolase	Test for the diagnosis of Wernicke's encephalopathy (WE); WE is a medical emergency, commonly occurring in alcoholics and others deficient in thiamine; presents with mental status changes sometimes associated with opthalmoplegia / ataxia
Toxicology screens	Multiple drugs can be screened for at once; useful for suspected drug misuse and for suspected overdoses of an unknown substance; specific drugs may also be requested
Heavy metal screens	Many neuropsychiatric symptoms have been associated with lead, mercury, manganese, arsenic and aluminum poisoning; these should be tested if a patient with psychiatric presentation has any suggestion of a history of exposure to them

Plasma Level Monitoring of Psychotropic and Antiepileptic Drugs

Monitoring plasma levels can assist in the overall treatment of the patient. However, blood tests are an inconvenience for both patients and staff, and drug assays add to laboratory time and costs. It is worthwhile knowing when and for which drugs plasma level monitoring is most useful. Situations when antiepileptic and psychotropic drug assays may be useful are:

◆   for monitoring patient concordance with drug therapy

◆   for optimising the drug treatment of certain disorders where a target range has been identified e.g. phenytoin for epilepsy, lithium for prophylaxis of bipolar affective disorder

◆   to confirm suspected toxicity, e.g. suspected lithium toxicity

◆   in deciding when to start drug therapy after an intentional overdose, e.g. tricyclic anti-depressants

◆   to confirm suspected drug interactions, or monitoring of potential drug interactions, e.g. using valproate and carbamazepine together

◆   monitoring drug levels in pregnancy and illness e.g. chronic liver disease

◆   when treating patients who have difficulty in reporting adverse effects, e.g. children, patients with learning disabilities or cognitive impairment.

The drugs for which plasma level monitoring is most informative should fulfil all of the following criteria:

◆   There is an accurate and specific assay method available.

◆   There is a large variation in the excretion or metabolism of the drug between individual patients.

◆   The clinical response to the drug is difficult to assess.

◆   The difference in plasma level between the therapeutic level and the toxic level is small (i.e. narrow therapeutic index).

◆   The drug has no active metabolites.

Of the psychotropics and antiepileptics, lithium and phenytoin are the only drugs that fulfil this criteria. However, plasma level monitoring of drugs that fulfil some of these criteria can still be useful. See Following Table.

It is worth noting that when a "target range" for a drug is quoted, it is an *average* range in which most patients respond.

For example:

A patient taking carbamazepine for epilepsy has a carbamazepine level of 8mg/L (therapeutic range = 4-12mg/L). The patient does not experience any side-effects but is still having frequent seizures. Although the carbamazepine level is "in the range" it is prudent to increase the dose of carbamazepine in light of the lack of efficacy.

The time at which the blood sample is taken in relation to when the tablets are taken is vital for the plasma level to be meaningful. Even once the drug levels in the body are at steady-state (i.e. 4-5 × half-life after start of therapy), plasma levels vary throughout the day. Generally it is best to take blood samples when the plasma levels are lowest (i.e. a trough level), for example, taking pre-dose carbamazepine levels (see Following Table). After the first sample it is best for subsequent samples to be taken at the same time. Apparent variations in plasma levels are often the result of sampling at different times. In particular, the widespread practice of withholding doses until a sample is taken is especially likely to provide a spurious result. All results should be compared with previous values so that anomalies can be detected.

Plasma Level Monitoring of Psychotropic and Antiepileptic Drugs

Drug	Sample Time (Time to Steady State)	Recommended Target Concentration	Comments
Carbamazepine	pre-dose (1-2 weeks – see comments)	4-12 mg/L (epilepsy) 7-12 mg/L (bipolar affective disorder – see comments)	Active metabolite. Auto-induction occurs; wait 2 weeks after target dose is reached before sampling. Levels >7mg/L are thought to be associated with efficacy for mania and bipolar affective disorder (Taylor & Duncan, 1997).
Clozapine	pre-dose (2-4 days)	clozapine >350 mcg/L (> 0.35mg/l)	Perry et al (1991) showed that patients were more likely to respond if the plasma level was >350mcg/l (64% vs 22%) and that 5 of 7 non responders became responders when their level was increased to >350mcg/l. Similar results were found by Potkin et al, 1994. See also Taylor and Duncan (1995).
Gabapentin	see comments	None	Plasma level monitoring is not currently recommended and the dose should be adjusted according to patient response.
Lamotrigine	see comments	None	Even though a recommended target concentration of 1-4mg/l has been suggested, a useful relationship has not been demonstrated between plasma concentration and effect or toxicity (Kilpatrick et al, 1996). The dose should be adjusted according to efficacy and tolerability.
Lithium	12 hours post-dose (5-7 days)	0.6-1.2 mmol/L	Plasma level monitoring should be done (minimum) weekly until target level reached, then monthly, then 3 monthly.
Olanzapine	see comments	None	A therapeutic range has not yet been defined but an accurate and specific assay has been developed (Aravagiri et al, 1997).

Phenobarbitone Primidone	pre-dose (2-3 weeks)	5-15 mg/L (primidone) 15-35 mg/L (phenobarbitone) 60-180 µmol/L (phenobarbitone)	As primidone is metabolised to phenobarbitone, it is essential to measure both levels in patients on primidone. Plasma levels may not be meaningful as tolerance develops.
Phenytoin	Pre-dose (2-14 days – dose dependent)	10-20 mg/L 40-80 µmols/L	Follows non-linear kinetics. Plasma level monitoring is essential. Highly protein bound, free levels are also useful.
Valproate	pre-dose – at a fixed time in relation to meals – see comments (2-5 days)	50-100 mg/L (bipolar affective disorder)	Levels >50mg/L are thought to be effective for mania and bipolar affective disorder. No clear correlation for seizure control. Diurnal variation also affected by free fatty acid concentration in plasma. Highly protein bound, free levels are also useful, but rarely measured.
SSRIs	see comments	None	Plasma levels are not thought to be useful. Test compliance only.
Topiramate	see comments	None	No clear correlation between trough plasma concentrations and therapeutic response has been established.
Tricyclic Antidepressants	see comments	Nortriptyline: 50-150 mcg/L (reference ranges for other tricyclics not as well established)	Most useful in suspected drug interactions or overdose and in people in whom there has been a poor response at normal doses.
Vigabatrin	see comments	None	No clear correlation between trough plasma concentrations and therapeutic response has been established.

Cerebrospinal Fluid Testing in Psychiatry

Cerebrospinal Fluid has many uses in psychiatry, but is predominantly used to rule out neurological disorders presenting with psychiatric symptoms. The following tables show the major indications and contraindications for this procedure.

Indications for Lumbar Puncture
modified from McConnell (1998) and McConnell and Bianchine (1994)

In adults:

◆ suspected infections or post-infectious illness (bacterial, tuberculous viral and fungal meningitis, aseptic meningitis, infectious polyneuritis, HIV and herpes simplex encephalitis, encephalitis of uncertain cause)

◆ multiple sclerosis (oligoclonal bands, IgG index and myelin basic protein most useful tests)

◆ intracranial haemmorrhage (better evaluated in the first instance with neuroimaging; CSF may be diagnostic for subarachnoid haemmorrhage even if neuroimaging is negative, however)

◆ meningeal malignancy (pleocytosis, – protein, – glucose, specific tumor markers)

◆ paraneoplastic syndromes (specific neuronal nuclear and Purkinje cell antibodies detectable)

◆ pseudotumor cerebri (requires lumbar puncture to diagnose)

◆ normal pressure hydrocephalus

◆ amyloid angiopathy (cystatin C, amyloid beta-protein)

◆ neurosarcoidosis (CSF angiotensin converting enzyme)

◆ evaluation of dementia (specific markers)

◆ stroke (where CNS vasculitis is suspected, if septic emboli suspected, in patients with positive syphilis or HIV serology, and in young patients with unexplained strokes)

◆ other (systemic lupus erythematosus, hepatic encephalopathy, vitamin B12 deficiency, occasionally in seizures to exclude CNS infection or bleed, and for intrathecal therapy)

In children:

◆ suspected meningitis (CSF changes may be less specific and initially normal in children)

◆ other infections (as with adults; most show non-specific changes except for antibody titers in SSPE, measles, rubella, and progressive rubella panencephalitis)

◆ febrile seizures – only if clinical evidence of meningitis is present, except in infants <12 months where clinical signs may be absent and CSF should be examined)

◆ intracranial haemmorhage in neonates

◆ pseudotumor cerebri

◆ lead encephalopathy

◆ CNS neoplasia (as with adults; best evaluated in the first instance with neuroimaging)

◆ lysosomal storage diseases (measurement of specific glycosphingolipids)

◆ therapeutic lumbar puncture (intrathecal therapy)

Contraindications to lumbar puncture
Modified from McConnell (1998) and McConnell and Bianchine (1994)

◆ if there is suspicion of increased intracranial pressure with a mass lesion or ventricular obstruction; in such instances neuroimaging should always be obtained first.

◆ in the presence of complete spinal subarachnoid block

◆ in the presence of notable coagulation defects

◆ if there is evidence of local infection at the site of the lumbar puncture in the case of known bacteraemia, one should be extra careful with lumbar puncture as it has been associated with the occurrence of secondary meningitis

CSF levels of various psychotropics are readily measured but are of research interest only at this time. The interested reader is referred to McConnell (1998) and McConnell and Bianchine (1994).

Electroencephalography (EEG) in Psychiatry

The EEG is a frequently used (and frequently misused!) tool in Psychiatry. The table below shows the common indications for its use in treating patients with psychiatric illness.

Indications For EEG in Psychiatry
Modified from McConnell (1998) and McConnell and Andrews (1999)

Indication	Comment
Suspected epilepsy	– Useful in the evaluation of episodic behavioural disorders e.g. atypical panic attacks, e.g. atypical paroxysmal affective or psychotic symptoms, rapid cycling, e.g. transient cognitive impairment or inattention in children – Sleep EEG and Ambulatory or video – EEG is often helpful – activation procedures are also useful – A normal EEG does not rule out epilepsy, nor does an abnormal EEG confirm it
Acute confusional states	– EEG is useful for both establishing the diagnosis and following the course of delirium
Other Cognitive Impairment	– EEG is useful in the diagnosis of dementia and of cognitive impairment related to depression or to medication effects
Other suspected neurological or medical illness presenting with psychiatric symptoms	– EEG indicated where findings in the history, mental state exam, physical exam or laboratory tests suggest a neurological or medical basis for the patient's symptoms **– EEG is not indicated for general screening of psychiatric patients or for the evaluation of primary psychiatric illness**
Electroconvulsive therapy (ECT)	– EEG monitoring useful to establish seizure duration during ECT
Suspected Drug Toxicity	– EEG is useful in evaluating suspected lithium and AED toxicity in patients who develop mental symptoms at therapeutic levels;

The EEG is affected by many psychotropics and this must always be considered when ordering this test. These are summarised in the following table:

EEG Changes Related to Treatment with Psychotropics

Modified from McConnell and Andrews (1999) and McConnell and Snyder (1998)

Drug	Within therapeutic range	In Overdose
Antipsychotics	– minor slowing of alpha – increased voltage of theta – clozapine may produce spike-wave complexes	– diffuse slowing – decreased alpha – occasionally increased sharp activity or spikes
Benzodiazepines	– increased beta activity	– diffuse slowing with superimposed beta activity
Lithium	– decreased amount and frequency of alpha activity	– diffuse slowing; decreased alpha; sharp waves
MAOIs	– usually none apparent	– diffuse slowing
SSRIs	– usually none apparent on visual inspection	– diffuse slowing – occasionally increased sharp activity or spikes
Stimulants	– increased beta and alpha activity	– diffuse slowing – sharp waves
Tricyclic Antidepressants	– increased theta and/or beta activity – occasionally decreased alpha	– diffuse slowing – may be superimposed beta activity

Monitoring of Drug Therapy

The clinical history is the most important measure of both the therapeutic effects and toxicity of psychotropics. Laboratory measure can, however, be of value in following the course of some psychotropics as outlined in the tables above. With the use of atypical psychotropics it is particularly important to follow certain laboratory parameters in addition to the usual clinical measures. These are outlined in the following table.

Monitoring Atypical

Drug	Obligatory Monitoring		Suggested Additional
	Baseline	Continuation	Baseline
Clozapine	FBC (Prescriber and pharmacist must register)	FBC – weekly for 18 weeks – at least fortnightly for first year – monthly thereafter	–ECG –EEG –LFTs –U&Es –BP –CPK –Temperature –Weight
Risperidone	None	None	–FBC –LFTs –U&Es –BP –Prolactin –CPK –Weight
Olanzapine	None	None	–FBC –LFTs –U&Es –BP –CPK –Weight –Prolactin
Quetiapine	None	None	–FBC –LFTs –BP –CPK –Weight –TFTs –U&Es
Amisulpride	None	None	–FBC –U&Es –CPK –Weight –Prolactin

KEY: –FBC Full blood count; –LFT Liver function tests; –ECG Electrocardiograph; –U&Es Urea & electrolytes

Modified from: Taylor D (1997). Monitoring the new antipsychotic drugs.

Antipsychotics

Monitoring	ACTIONS
Continuation	
ECG – when maintenance dose is reached. EEG – as above and if myoclonus or seizures occur. BP – 4-hourly during initiation. LFT/U&E – every 3-6 months. CPK – if NMS suspected. Temperature – daily for first 3 weeks, then weekly. Weight – as needed	**Stop** clozapine if neutrophil count below 1.5×10^9/L. Refer to specialist care if neutrophils below 0.5×10^9/L **Stop** clozapine if LFTs indicate hepatitis or reduced hepatic function (PT). Use Valproate if EEG shows clear epileptiform changes or if seizures occur. **Stop** clozapine if ECG changes or signs of heart failure. Monitor closely if temperature ↑.
FBC – 3-6 monthly LFTs – 3-6 monthly U&Es – 3-6 monthly BP – frequently during initiation. Prolactin – if symptoms occur. CPK – if NMS suspected Weight – as needed	**Stop** risperidone if neutrophils below 1.5×10^9/L. Use with caution in hepatic or renal failure. **Stop** risperidone if prolactin related effects intolerable. **Stop** risperidone if NMS suspected.
FBC – 3-6 monthly LFTs – monthly for 3 months U&Es – 3-6 monthly BP – frequently during initiation. CPK – if NMS suspected. Prolactin – if symptoms occur. Weight – as needed	**Stop** olanzapine if alkaline phosphatase, PT or bilirubin changed. **Stop** olanzapine if NMS suspected. **Stop** olanzapine if neutrophils below 1.5×10^9/L.
FBC – 3-6 monthly LFTs – monthly for 3 months BP -frequently during initiation CPK – if NMS suspected Weight – as needed TFTs – 3 monthly U&Es – 3-6 monthly	**Stop** quetiapine if alkaline phosphatase, PT or bilirubin change. **Stop** quetiapine if NMS suspected. **Stop** quetiapine if neutrophils below 1.5×10^9/L.
FBC – 3-6 monthly U&Es -3-6 monthly CPK – if NMS suspected Weight – as needed Prolactin – if symptoms occur	**Stop** amisulpride if neutrophils below 1.5×10^9/L **Stop** amisulpride if NMS suspected **Stop** amisulpride if prolactin related effects intolerable

– EEG	Electro-encephalograph	– BP	Blood Pressure
– CPK	Creatinine Phosphokinase	– TFT's	Thyroid Function Tests

II

Treatment of

Psychosis

Antipsychotics – General Principles of Prescribing

Aims

To ensure quality of prescribing of all antipsychotics and to shift the spectrum of use of novel antipsychotics from difficult to treat patients (for which only clozapine is indicated) to patients in earlier phases of illness.

Standards

◇ Each patient should ideally be prescribed only one antipsychotic, preferably in a single dosage form. (An exception is when switching from one drug to another.)

◇ Typical antipsychotics should ideally not be used as "PRN" sedatives. (Short courses of benzodiazepines or general sedatives (e.g. promethazine) may be used.)

◇ The lowest possible effective dose should be used, with patients given a sufficient trial on low doses before any further dose increases. This applies to both typical and atypical antipsychotics.

◇ *As a consequence*, doses above 15mg/day haloperidol or equivalent should be the exception rather than the rule. Patients receiving higher doses without resolution of symptoms should be considered for clozapine.

◇ Patients receiving >1g equivalent chlorpromazine should be monitored as outlined by the Royal College of Psychiatrists. Those showing a measured response should have this documented in their notes. Those not responding should be considered for clozapine.

◇ Anticholinergic drugs should be given for Parkinsonism or dystonia (prophylactically as necessary) but withdrawal should be attempted after 2-3 months without symptoms. Anticholinergics are liable to misuse and impair memory.

◇ Individual *atypical* antipsychotics should be used only for the indications outlined in the table *Indications for Atypical Drugs.*

Antipsychotic Drugs –

Drug	Chemical Group	Dose Range (daily dose) Single daily dose unless stated (*)	Alternative Indications
Chlorpromazine	Phenothiazine (Grp I – aliphatic)	25-1000mg	Anxiety, nausea, agitation, hiccup, induction of hypothermia, violence, autism.
Promazine	Phenothiazine (Grp I – aliphatic)	400-800mg	Agitation and restlessness in the elderly. **NB.** Weak antipsychotic.
Thioridazine	Phenothiazine (Grp II – piperidine)	150-800mg	Agitation, anxiety, violence, impulsive behaviour. Agitation and restlessness in the elderly.
Fluphenazine	Phenothiazine (Grp III – piperazine)	1-20mg	Agitation, anxiety, violence.
Perphenazine	Phenothiazine (Grp III – piperazine)	12-24mg	Agitation, severe anxiety, violence.
Trifluoperazine	Phenothiazine (Grp III – piperazine)	10-50mg (est.) (maximum dose not stated by manufacturers)	Agitation, severe anxiety, violence.
Flupenthixol	Thioxanthine	6-18mg	Depressive illness (lower doses).
Zuclopenthixol	Thioxanthine	20-150mg	None
Haloperidol	Butyrophenone	1.5-120mg	Agitation, severe anxiety, violence, tics, nausea, hiccup, mania, Gilles de la Tourette.
Droperidol	Butyrophenone	20-120mg (*QDS)	Anaesthesia, mania, nausea. **NB.** For acute (sedative) treatment only.
Benperidol	Butyrophenone	0.25-1.5mg (*BD)	Deviant social/sexual behaviour. **NB.** Not licensed for schizophrenia

Brief details (1)

Adverse Effects (See data sheet for full details/ section VII for comparison)	Interactions (See manufacturers' data for full information)	Cost
Extrapyramidal effects, anticholinergic effects, sedation, hypotension, hypothermia, endocrine disorders, convulsions, jaundice, ECG changes, blood dyscrasias	Sedatives, lithium, anticholinergics, antiepileptics, sulphonylureas, cimetidine, antidepressants, dopamine (ant)agonists	+
As chlorpromazine	As chlorpromazine	+
As chlorpromazine + pigmented retinopathy, ejaculatory dysfunction.	As chlorpromazine	+
As chlorpromazine + depression reported.	As chlorpromazine	+
As chlorpromazine.	As chlorpromazine	+
As chlorpromazine	As chlorpromazine	+
As chlorpromazine	As chlorpromazine	+
As chlorpromazine	As chlorpromazine	+
As chlorpromazine	As chlorpromazine + fluoxetine, carbamazepine, astemizole, terfenadine	+
As chlorpromazine + depression	As chlorpromazine	++
As chlorpromazine	As chlorpromazine	++

Antipsychotic Drugs –

Drug	Chemical Group	Dose Range (daily dose) Single daily dose unless stated (*)	Alternative Indications
Sulpiride	Substituted benzamide	400 – 2400mg (*BD)	None
Pimozide	Diphenylbutylpiperidine	2-20mg	Mania, hypochondriacal psychosis
Loxapine	Dibenzoxazepine	20-250mg (*BD)	None
Risperidone	Benzisoxazole	2-16mg	None
Olanzapine	Thienobenzodiazepine	5-20 mg/day	None
Quetiapine	Dibenzothiazepine	150-750mg (*BD) Lower doses in the elderly	None
Amisulpride	Substituted benzamide	Positive symptoms 400-1200mg (*BD) Negative Symptoms: 50-300mg	None
Clozapine See data sheet for restrictions to licence	Dibenzodiazepine	25-900mg (*BD or more frequently)	None

Brief details (2)

Adverse Effects (See data sheet for full details/ section VII for comparison)	Interactions (See manufacturers' data for full information)	Cost
As chlorpromazine, jaundice & skin reactions less common. Less sedation, hypotension	As chlorpromazine	++
As chlorpromazine + serious cardiac arrhythmias (monitor plasma potassium), depression	As chlorpromazine + diuretics, any cardioactive drug – this includes other antipsychotics and tricyclics	+
As chlorpromazine + nausea, dyspnoea, ptosis, polydipsia, paraesthesia	As chlorpromazine	++
Agitation, hypotension, abdominal pain, fatigue, anxiety, nausea, rhinitis, weight gain, etc. EPS uncommon with doses below 8mg/day. Prolactin changes may cause sexual dysfunction, etc	As chlorpromazine	+++
Sedation, weight gain, hypotension, anticholinergic effects, changes in LFTs	Smoking and carbamazepine reduce olanzapine levels to small extent	+++
Hypotension, sedation, dry mouth, constipation, weight gain, dizziness, LFT changes, TFT changes	Caution with potent inhibitors of CYP3A4. (e.g. ketoconazole/ nefazodone)	+++
Insomnia, agitation, anxiety, weight gain, extrapyramidal adverse effects, hyper-prolactinaemia, sedation	Few known interactions. Caution with other sedatives, including alcohol; dopamine agonists; and possibly hypotensives	+++
As chlorpromazine + hypersalivation, delirium, incontinence, myocarditis, neutropenia, fatal agranulocytosis (see table)	As chlorpromazine + all drugs which depress leucopoiesis: eg cytotoxic agents, sulphonamides, chloramphenicol, carbamazepine, phenothiazines. SSRIs (not citalopram) and risperidone increase clozapine plasma levels. Smoking, carbamazepine and phenytoin decrease clozapine levels.	++++

Algorithm for the Drug Treatment of Schizophrenia

(This represents an ideal scenario and may not always apply)

Give atypical antipsychotic at minimum effective dose.
Evaluate over six weeks; after titration, increase dose every two weeks (or longer) only if necessary.

* Non-adherence is common, especially if patients do not collaborate in their choice of treatment.

* Use benzodiazepines or promethazine if sedation or behavioural control are required. Short term use only (less than 4-6 weeks)

→ *Effective* / *Tolerated* → **Continue with oral therapy as sole antipsychotic**

Ineffective or partly effective / *Not tolerated*

↓

Change to a different antipsychotic.
Consider: typical drugs; amisulpride, olanzapine or risperidone for negative symptoms; quetiapine or olanzapine for EPS; quetiapine or olanzapine for symptomatic hyperprolactinaemia.
Evaluate over 6-8 weeks

Assess efficacy with recognised rating scales. e.g. BPRS, CGI

→ *Effective* / *Tolerated* → **Continue with oral therapy as sole antipsychotic**

Poor compliance

↓

Change to depot.
Use lowest known therapeutic dose at maximum allowable interval (unless practical issues demand otherwise). Adjust dose only at 2-3 month intervals.

* Consider augmentation strategies, e.g. lithium for schizoaffective disorder; carbamazepine for aggression; valproate for mood disturbance.

→ *Effective* / *Tolerated* → **Continue with depot as sole antipsychotic**

Ineffective (dashed line back)

* Consider compliance therapy as alternative to depot.

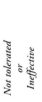

"Unproven therapies" if used, must be carefully evaluated using recognised rating scales over a prospectively fixed period (suggest 6-8 weeks). If possible, gain patient consent and document in notes.

Not tolerated or Ineffective

Change to clozapine.
Titrate slowly to 300-400mg/day and then by 25-50mg increments to give a plasma level above 350mcg/L.

Assess over at least six months.

Effective

Tolerated

If measured improvement, continue at same dose, as sole antipsychotic

Ineffective

Not tolerated

Consider unproven therapies
* Add sulpiride to clozapine.
* Clozapine with small doses of risperidone, haloperidol or amisulpride.
* High dose olanzapine (60mg/day)
* Omega - 3 marine triglycerides 5G BD
* ECT
* Add nefazodone?

Effective

Tolerated

If clearly measured improvement, continue and document in patient notes

Notes on Schizophrenia Algorithm

- The algorithm represents an ideal, evidence-based approach to the treatment of schizophrenia and related psychoses.
- It is assumed that no financial constraints influence drug choice. Where funding is capped or where the use of atypical antipsychotics is restricted to a fixed number of patients, the use of atypicals first-line may be inappropriate.
- Low dose typical antipsychotics may be used first-line where financial restrictions apply. For example, haloperidol 2-4mg/day can be an effective, well-tolerated regimen. Ideally, atypicals are preferred because of their proven low incidence of extrapyramidal adverse effects, their lack of effect on serum prolactin (not amisulpride or risperidone), and their superior activity against negative symptoms (not quetiapine).
- There is no firm evidence that any drug except clozapine is effective in refractory schizophrenia. Clozapine should be used where two antipsychotics have failed (not more). Note that the longer the duration of poorly treated illness, the worse the prognosis.

Advice on Prescribing Depot Medication

Give a test dose

Depots are long-acting. Any adverse effects which result from injection are likely to be long-lived. Thus a small test dose is essential to avoid severe, prolonged adverse effects. See table and manufacturer's information.

Begin with the lowest therapeutic dose

There are few data showing clear dose-response effects for depot preparations. There is some information which indicates that low doses are at least as effective as higher ones. Low doses are likely to be better tolerated and are certainly less expensive.

Administer at the longest possible licensed interval

All depots can be safely administered at their licensed dosing intervals. There is no evidence to suggest that shortening the dose interval improves efficacy. Moreover, injections are painful, so less frequent administration is desirable. The "observation" that some patients deteriorate in the days before the next depot is due is probably fallacious. For some hours (or even days with some preparations) plasma levels of antipsychotics continue to fall, albeit slowly, after the next injection. Thus patients are most at risk of deterioration immediately after a depot injection and not before it. Moreover, in trials, relapse seems only to occur 3-6 months after withdrawing depot therapy; roughly the time required to clear steady-state depot drug levels from the blood.

Adjust doses only after an adequate period of assessment

Attainment of peak plasma levels, therapeutic effect and steady state plasma levels are all delayed with depot injections. Doses may be reduced if adverse effects occur, but should only be increased after careful assessment over at least one month, preferably longer. The use of adjunctive oral medication to assess depot requirements may be helpful, but it too is complicated by the slow emergence of antipsychotic effects. Note that at the start of therapy, plasma levels of antipsychotic released from a depot increase over several weeks without increasing the given dose. Dose increases during this time to steady state plasma levels are thus illogical and impossible properly to evaluate.

Antipsychotic Depot Injections

Suggested doses and frequencies

Drug	Trade Name	Test Dose (mg)	Dose Range (mg / week)	Dosing Interval (weeks)	Comments
Flupenthixol decanoate	*Depixol*	20	12.5- 400	2 – 4	? Mood elevating; may worsen agitation
Fluphenazine decanoate	*Modecate*	12.5	6.25 – 50	2 – 5	Avoid in depression. High EPS
Haloperidol decanoate	*Haldol*	25*	12.5 – 75	4	High EPS, low incidence of sedation
Pipothiazine palmitate	*Piportil*	25	12.5 – 50	4	? Lower incidence of EPS
Zuclopenthixol decanoate	*Clopixol*	100	100 – 600	2 – 4	? Useful in agitation and aggression

Notes

● Give a quarter or half stated doses in elderly.

● After test dose, wait 4-10 days before starting titration to maintenance therapy (see product information for individual drugs)

● Dose range is given in mg/week for convenience only – avoid using shorter dose intervals than those recommended except in exceptional circumstances eg. long interval necessitates high volume (>3-4ml) injection.

● EPS = extrapyramidal side effects.

* Test dose not stated by manufacturer

Modified from Taylor D, Duncan D, 1995.
Antipsychotic depot injections – suggested doses and frequencies.
Psychiatric Bulletin; 19, 357.

Clozapine – Dosing Regimen

Many of clozapine's adverse effects are dose-dependent and are possibly associated with a rapid increase in dose. Adverse effects also tend to be more common at the beginning of therapy. To minimise these problems it is important to start therapy at a low dose and to increase slowly.

Clozapine should be started at a dose of 12.5 mg once a day. Blood pressure should be monitored hourly for six hours because of clozapine's hypotensive effect. This monitoring is not usually necessary if the first dose is given at night. On day two, the dose can be increased to 12.5 mg twice daily. If the patient is tolerating the clozapine, the dose can then be increased by 25 mg to 50 mg a day, until a dose of 300mg a day is reached. This can usually be achieved in two to three weeks.

Further dosage increases should be made slowly in increments of 50 mg to 100 mg each week. A dose of 450mg/day or a plasma level of 350mcg/L should be aimed for. The total clozapine dose should be divided and, if sedation is a problem, the larger portion of the dose can be given at night.

The following table is a suggested starting regime for clozapine. This is a cautious regimen – more rapid increases have been used in exceptional circumstances. Slower titration may be necessary where sedation is severe.

Day	Morning Dose	Evening Dose
1	–	12.5
2	12.5	12.5
3	25	25
4	25	25
5	25	50
6	25	50
7	50	50
8	50	75
9	75	75
10	75	100
11	100	100
12	100	125
13	125	125
14	125	150
15	150	150
18	150	200
21	200	200
28	200	250

If the patient is not tolerating a particular dose, decrease to one which was being tolerated. If the adverse effect resolves, increase the dose again but at a slower rate. If for any reason a patient misses *less than* two day's clozapine, restart at the dose prescribed before the event. Do not administer extra tablets to catch up. If more than two days are missed: restart at 12.5mg once daily and increase slowly (but at a faster rate than in drug-naive patients).

31

Indications for Atypical Drugs

Assuming no financial restraint

Indication	1st choice(s)	Alternatives
❖ 1st episode psychosis and acute relapse	Any atypical (not clozapine)	
❖ Symptomatic, uncontrolled acute extrapyramidal effects or prior dystonic reaction	Olanzapine Quetiapine	Risperidone (low dose)
❖ Symptomatic, uncontrolled hyperprolactinaemia	Olanzapine Quetiapine	None
❖ Predominant, unresponsive negative symptoms	Olanzapine Risperidone Amisulpride	Clozapine
❖ Treatment-refractory psychosis (including patients intolerant of typical antipsychotics)	Clozapine	None
❖ Physically or socially disabling tardive dyskinesia	Clozapine	None
❖ Ongoing neuro-cognitive or rehabilitation disability on typical or atypical drug	Clozapine	None

Atypical Antipsychotics – Titration Details

Drug	Starting dose	Minimum effective dose	Maximum dose (may differ from manufacturer's recommendations)
Clozapine (See table)	12.5 mg/day	around 300 mg/day (lower in elderly)	900 mg/day
Olanzapine	10 mg/day (5 mg in some – see product literature)	5 – 10 mg/day	20 mg/day (ceiling dose not yet defined)
Risperidone	2 mg/day (1 mg in elderly)	4 mg/day ? lower in some (e.g. elderly)	8 mg/day (higher doses should be avoided)
Quetiapine	50 mg/day (25 mg in elderly)	300 mg/day (? lower in elderly)	750 mg/day (but no evidence of improved efficacy over 300 mg/day)
Amisulpride	800 mg/day	800 mg/day for positive symptoms. 100 mg/day for negative symptoms.	1200 mg/day (but no evidence of improved efficacy over 800 mg)

Recommended procedure:

Introduce drug Titrate to lowest effective dose
Add sedative for behavioural control if required Evaluate over at least two weeks

 No response

Stop drug if insufficient response at maximum dose for two or more weeks Repeat evaluations and increments as necessary Increase dose by 25 -50% or according to manufacturer's recommendations

Atypical Antipsychotics – Minimising Costs

Atypical antipsychotics are relatively costly medicines, although their benefits may make them cost effective in practice. Cost minimisation is a practical option which reduces drug expenditure without compromising patient care or patient quality of life. It involves using the right drug for the most appropriate condition (see Protocols) and using the minimum effective dose in each patient. A guide to what is likely to be the minimum effective dose can be obtained from clinical trials using fixed doses or fixed ranges of doses of atypicals. The table below gives the cost (£/patient/30 days) in January 1999 of atypicals at their lowest effective dose, their approximate average clinical dose, and their licensed maximum dose. The table allows comparison of different doses of the same drug and of different drugs at any of the three doses. It is hoped that the table will encourage the use of lower doses of less expensive drugs, given equality in other respects and allowing for clinical need.

Atypic Drugs – Costs

Drug	Minimum effective dose cost [1]	Approximate clinical average dose cost [1,2]	Maximum dose cost [1]
Clozapine N.B. No alternative available for refractory schizophrenia	Not known – too variable	450 mg/day £241.32	900 mg/day £482.63
Risperidone	4 mg/day £77.22	6 mg/day £117.00	16 mg/day £308.88
Olanzapine	10 mg/day £113.00	15 mg/day £169.50	20 mg/day £226.00
Quetiapine	300 mg/day £113.10	500 mg/day £169.65	750 mg/day £254.40
Amisulpride	400 mg/day (?)[3] £60.00	800 mg/day £120.00	1200 mg/day £180.00

1) Costs are for UK adults (for 30 days) MIMS January 1999.
2) Average clinical doses are for adult inpatients in maintenance therapy (Taylor D. et al., 1999).
3) Dose depends on target symptoms.

Treatment of Acute Relapse of Psychosis

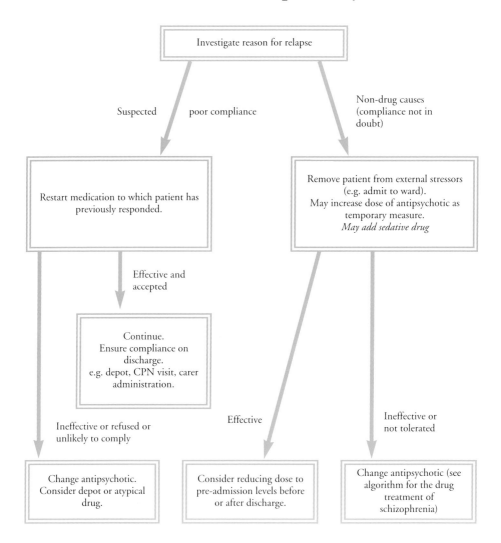

Investigate reason for relapse

Suspected   poor compliance

Non-drug causes (compliance not in doubt)

Restart medication to which patient has previously responded.

Remove patient from external stressors (e.g. admit to ward).
May increase dose of antipsychotic as temporary measure.
May add sedative drug

Effective and accepted

Continue.
Ensure compliance on discharge.
e.g. depot, CPN visit, carer administration.

Ineffective or refused or unlikely to comply

Effective

Ineffective or not tolerated

Change antipsychotic.
Consider depot or atypical drug.

Consider reducing dose to pre-admission levels before or after discharge.

Change antipsychotic (see algorithm for the drug treatment of schizophrenia)

*Other reasons for relapse include mood disturbance and violence. Refer to specific protocols.

Equivalent Doses of Antipsychotics

Drug	Equivalent Dose (Consensus) (mg/ day)	Range of Values in literature (mg/ day)
Chlorpromazine	100	-
Thioridazine	100	75 – 100
Fluphenazine	2	2 – 5
Trifluoperazine	5	2.5 – 5
Flupenthixol	3	2 – 3
Zuclopenthixol	25	25 – 60
Haloperidol	3	1.5 – 5
Droperidol	4	1 – 4
Sulpiride	200	200 – 270
Pimozide	2	2
Loxapine	10	10 – 25
Fluphenazine *depot*	5/ week	1 – 12.5/ week
Pipothiazine *depot*	10/ week	10 – 12.5/ week
Flupenthixol *depot*	10/ week	10 – 20/ week
Zuclopenthixol *depot*	100/ week	40 – 100/ week
Haloperidol *depot*	15/ week	5 – 25/ week

Note – all values should be regarded as approximate
Dose equivalencies are not relevant to atypical drugs:
therapeutic doses are well defined.

Antipsychotics Maximum Doses

DRUG	MAXIMUM DOSE (mg/day)
Chlorpromazine	1000
Thioridazine	800 (see BNF)
Fluphenazine	20
Trifluoperazine	None (suggest 50)
Flupenthixol	18
Zuclopenthixol	150
Haloperidol	120
Droperidol	120
Sulpiride	2400
Pimozide	20
Loxapine	250
Clozapine	900
Risperidone	16
Amisulpride	1200
Olanzapine	20
Fluphenazine *depot*	50/week
Pipothiazine *depot*	50/week
Haloperidol *depot*	300 every 4 weeks
Flupenthixol *depot*	400/week
Zuclopenthixol *depot*	600/week

Note

Doses above these maxima should only be used in extreme circumstances: there is no evidence for improved efficacy. Always follow RCP guidelines.

Oral / Parenteral Dose Equivalents

DRUG	ORAL DOSE (mg)	EQUIVALENT IM OR IV DOSE (mg)
Antipsychotics		
Chlorpromazine	100	25-50*
Droperidol	10	7.5
Haloperidol	10	5
Promazine	100	100
Anticholinergics		
Procyclidine	10	7.5

Note

Because of the variation in bioavailability with some drugs, prescriptions should always specify the dose and a single route of administration.

For example:

Droperidol 10mg IM Q6H PRN

* IM/IV chlorpromazine not recommended

III

Treatment of
Affective Illness

Antidepressant Drugs

Tricyclic	Main Indication	Alternative Indications (#Not Licensed)	Dosing	Adverse Effects/ Contraindications
Amitriptyline	Depression	Enuresis in children Migraine prophylaxis# Anxiolytic#	25-150mg/day (once daily) child > 7 yrs 10-20mg daily	Sedation, often with hangover; postural hypotension; tachycardia/ arrhythmias; Dry mouth, blurred vision, constipation, retention C/I: Prostatism, narrow angle glaucoma, post MI, heart block. Caution in epilepsy, liver disease.
Nortriptyline	Depression	As for amitriptyline	20-150 mg once daily	As for amitriptyline, but less sedative, less anticholinergic, no postural hypotension
Dothiepin	Depression	None	75-225mg once daily	As for amitriptyline
Imipramine	Depression	As for amitriptyline	75-200 mg 300 mg max in inpatients once daily	As for amitriptyline, but less sedative
Desipramine	Depression	None	75-200 mg once daily	As for nortriptyline, Hypotension may occur
Clomipramine	Depression	Obsessive comp- ulsive disorder Phobic states Cataplexy associated with narcolepsy	10-250 mg once daily	As for amitriptyline
Lofepramine	Depression	None	70-210mg/day BD or TDS	As amitriptyline, but less sedative/anticholinergic/ cardiotoxic
Trimipramine	Depression	None	75-300 mg once daily	As for amitriptyline, but more sedative

– Tricyclics

Interactions	Half Life (hrs)	Cost (&)	Comments
Alcohol Anticholinergics (inc neuroleptics, etc) MAOIs Sympathomimetics Cimetidine	8-24	0.02 / 50mg	Due to long $t_{1/2}$,SR preparations unnecessary Metabolised to nortriptyline Liquid form available
As for amitriptyline	18-96	0.10 / 25mg	Good <u>mildly</u> sedating antidepressant; particularly useful in the elderly.
As for amitriptyline	11-40	0.14 / 75mg	Very similar to amitriptyline: structure only differs by replacing C with S atom in tricyclic ring. Very dangerous in overdose. Liquid form available
As for amitriptyline	4-18	0.04 / 25mg	Metabolised to desipramine. Liquid form available
As for amitriptyline	12-24	0.04 / 25mg	Not currently marketed in UK but widely used elsewhere
As for amitriptyline	17-28	0.14 / 50mg	Liquid form available
As for amitriptyline	1.5-6	0.18 / 70mg	Metabolised to desipramine. <u>Safer in overdose</u> Liquid available
As for amitriptyline Safer with MAOIs than other tricyclics	7-23	0.18 / 50mg	Most sedating antidepressant

Antidepressant Drugs

SSRIs	Main Indication	Alternative Indications (#Not Licensed)	Dosing	Adverse Effects/ Contraindications
Fluvoxamine	Depression	OCD	100-300mg/day BD if > 100mg	Nausea, diarrhoea, agitation, insomnia, dry mouth & blurred vision, tremor, dizziness, hyponatraemia, sexual dysfunction (male and female). Somnolence may occur rarely Caution in epilepsy
Fluoxetine	Depression – including that associated with anxiety	Bulimia, OCD	20 mg /day (depression)60 mg /day (bulimia) 20-60mg/day (OCD)	As fluvoxamine, but: weight loss and rash may occur. Insomnia and agitation possibly more common. Hypoglycaemia may occur rarely: avoid in diabetes. Vasculitis may occur very rarely.
Sertraline	Depression – including that associated with anxiety	Preventing relapse of depressive illness	50 -100 mg once daily 150-200 mg/day may be used for eight weeks only	As fluvoxamine, but: sexual dysfunction may be more common, nausea less common. Contra-indicated in hepatic failure, caution in renal failure
Paroxetine	Depression – including that associated with anxiety	OCD Panic Disorder +/- agoraphobia Social phobia	20-50mg/day (depression) 20-60mg/day (OCD) 10-50mg/day (panic disorder)	As fluvoxamine, but: sedation more likely. Extra-pyramidal symptoms more common, but rare. Withdrawal effects common
Citalopram	Depression	Preventing relapse of depressive illness Panic disorder +/- agoraphobia	20 – 60mg once daily	As fluvoxamine, but: nausea may be less common

– SSRIs

Interactions	Half-Life (hrs)	Cost (£)	Comments
Inhibits hepatic demethylation: (CYP1A2). Caution with TCAs, warfarin, phenytoin, clozapine theophylline; MAOIs never. Care with lithium, tryptophan, alcohol.	15 single dose 17-22 multiple dose	0.63 / 100mg	Safe in overdose (this applies to all SSRIs). Relatively high incidence of nausea reported in some trials and observed in clinical practice.
As fluvoxamine but safe with theophylline. Inhibits CYP2D6, CYP3A4. MAOIs / tryptophan never. Increases plasma levels of tricyclics, benzos, clozapine and cyclosporin. No interaction with alcohol.	24-140	0.69 / 20mg	Undoubted efficacy but not useful where degree of sedation is required. Active metabolite has $t_{1/2}$ of 7-9 days. Wide range of interactions reported. Liquid form available.
As fluvoxamine but safe with theophylline. Inhibits CYP2D6. Care with lithium/ tryptophan, alcohol. MAOIs never. Alcohol – caution.	24-26	0.95 / 100mg	Less potent inhibitor of CYP2D6 but some interactions reported
As fluoxetine. Safe with theophylline and alcohol. Inhibits CYP2D6. MAOIs never.	24	0.69 / 20mg	No active metabolites. Withdrawal reaction more frequently reported – withdraw very slowly. Liquid form available.
Few interactions reported. MAOIs never. Safe with alcohol.	33	0.60 / 20mg	Poor inhibitor of CYP2D6 and so may cause fewer adverse drug interactions.

Antidepressant Drugs

MAOIs	Main Indication	Alternative Indications (#Not Licensed)	Dosing	Adverse Effects/ Contraindications
Phenelzine	Depressive illness where phobic symptoms are present	Anxiety states# Obsessive compulsive disorder#	15-30 mg tds	Anticholinergic effects Nervousness Weight gain, hypotension Hepatotoxicity, oedema Leucopenia Psychosis CI: CVS disease, Phaeochromocytoma Liver disease Diabetes
Tranyl-cypromine	As for phenelzine	As for phenelzine	10 mg b.d. Max. 30mg/day BD total dose before mid pm	As for phenelzine but even more caution required Additionally, hyperthyroidism, insomnia Hepatotoxicity and weight gain less common
Isocarboxazid	As for phenelzine	As for phenelzine	30-60 mg loading for six weeks 10-20 mg maintenance once daily	As for phenelzine but may cause weight loss, more hepatotoxicity, less hypotension
Moclobemide	Major depressive illness	None	300-600mg/day BD after food Last dose before 3.00pm	Insomnia, nausea, agitation, confusion Hypertension reported – may be related to tyramine ingestion

– MAOIs

Interactions	Half- Life (hrs)	Cost (£)	Comments
Tyramine in food Always carry an MAOI card Sympathomimetics Opioids Tricyclics Tryptophan SSRIs Venlafaxine	1.5	0.07 / 15mg	Phenelzine is possibly the safest of MAOI's and is the one that should be used if combinations are being considered
As for phenelzine, only more severe and never with tricyclics	2.5	0.05 / 10mg	Mild dependence, amphetamine-like structure ? metabolised to amphetamine. More potent adverse effects, never use in combination
As for phenelzine	36	0.05 / 10mg	Similar to phenelzine except longer half-life.
Tyramine interactions rare and mild Opioid interactions limited to pethidine and ? codeine Avoid: sympathomimetics, SSRIs, clomipramine, l-dopa Caution: TCAs, lithium, sumatriptan Cimetidine – use half dose of moclobemide	1-2	0.35/ 150mg	Reversible inhibitor of MAOI-A. Fewer adverse effects, fewer drug interactions. Food interactions possible if high doses (>600mg/day) used or if large quantities of tyramine ingested.

Antidepressant Drugs

Drug	Main Indication	Alternative Indications	Dosing	Adverse Effects / Contraindications
Trazodone	Depression	None	150-600mg/day once daily (bd above 300mg)	As amitriptyline, but not anticholinergic, less cardiotoxic
Nefazodone	Depression	None	200-600 mg/day (BD)	As trazodone, but less sedative, less hypotensive
Venlafaxine	Depressive illness	None	75-375 daily (BD) after food XL prep is OD, max dose 225mg/ day	Nausea, insomnia, dry mouth, sexual dysfunction., drowsiness, headache. Elevation of blood pressure at higher doses. Discontinue if rash occurs. Halve dose in hepatic/renal impairment. Withdrawal effects are common even if doses are a few hours late.
Reboxetine	Treatment of depression and maintenance of improvement	None, but limited data to suggest reboxetine improves social functioning	8-12mg/day (BD)	Insomnia, sweating, dizziness, dry mouth, constipation, urinary hesitation.
Mirtazapine	Depression	None	15-45mg/day As single dose at night	Drowsiness (low dose), increased appetite, weight gain. Rarely, blood dyscrasias, LFT changes, convulsions, myoclonus, oedema.

– Others

Interactions	Half Life (hrs)	Cost	Comments
As amitriptyline but safer in epilepsy.	1-13	0.36 / 100mg	Sedative, not anticholinergic. Priapism possible. Liquid available.
Potent inhibitor of CYP3A4. See Data Sheet.	2 – 4	0.30/200mg	Sexual dysfunction rarely reported.
Few reported Care with lithium MAOIs – never Care with cimetidine Minor effect on CYP enzymes	5 (11 for active metabolite)	0.72/75mg	Limited data to support special properties of venlafaxine: fast onset; greater efficacy; efficacy in refractory illness. Further studies/clinical experience needed to confirm or refute these.
Information is incomplete. Minor effect on CYP2D6/3A4. MAOIs – never No interaction with alcohol.	13	0.33/ 4mg tab	Impotence is rare, occurs mainly in men and is dose-related. Safe in overdose
Minimal effect on CYP2D6/1A2/3A. Avoid with other sedatives including alcohol. MAOIs – never.	20-40	0.86/ 30mg tab	Appears safe in overdose, sexual dysfunction is rare.

Algorithm for the Drug Treatment of Depression

Give therapeutic dose of antidepressant

Assess over at least four weeks

→ Effective/Tolerated → Continue at therapeutic dose for six months #

Withdraw slowly

Not tolerated

Ineffective
(Check compliance)

↓

Change to different class of antidepressant at therapeutic dose

Assess over at least four weeks

→ Effective/Tolerated → Continue at therapeutic doses for six months #

Withdraw slowly

Not tolerated

Ineffective

↓

Lithium augmentation
Add lithium to level > 0.4mmol/l

Assess over at least three weeks

→ Effective/Tolerated → Continue at therapeutic doses for six months #

Withdraw slowly

Not tolerated

Ineffective
(withdraw lithium)

↓

Augment with electro-convulsive therapy
6-12 treatments

Usually abandon after 8 treatments if no response

→ Effective/Tolerated → Continue with antidepressant at therapeutic doses for 6 months #

Withdraw slowly

Not tolerated

Ineffective

↓

49

Augment with liothyronine (T₃)
20-50mcg/day

Assess over four weeks

Effective/ Tolerated →

Continue at therapeutic doses for six months +
Monitor TFTs
Withdraw slowly

Ineffective   Not tolerated

Consider other putative treatments*

Examples include:

Venlafaxine (high dose)
TCA (high dose) – with ECG monitoring
TCA + SSRI (TCA must be low dose)
MAOI + TCA (e.g. trimipramine + phenelzine)
SSRI + pindolol 5mg TDS
Dexamethasone augmentation (3mg/day for 4 days)
SSRI + buspirone 20-30mg/ day

Effective/ Tolerated →

Continue for at least six months (not dexamethasone)
Monitor TCA levels when used at high dose or with SSRI

Withdraw slowly

* Only limited evidence to support these combinations – few well-controlled, prospective, randomised studies.
# Consider life-long treatment in recurrent depression.

Antidepressants – Swapping and Stopping

General guidelines

1. All antidepressants have the potential to cause withdrawal phenomena. When taken continuously for six weeks or longer, antidepressants should not be stopped abruptly unless a serious adverse effect has occurred (e.g. cardiac arrhythmia with a tricyclic).

2. Antidepressants should be withdrawn slowly, preferably over four weeks, by weekly decrements.

Examples:		Decrements			
Drug	**Maintenance dose** (mg/day)	**Dose after 1st** (mg/day)	**Dose after 2nd** (mg/day)	**Dose after 3rd** (mg/day)	**Dose after 4th** (mg/day)
Amitriptyline	150	100	50	25	Nil
Paroxetine	30	20	10	10mg alt die	Nil
Trazodone	450	300	150	75	Nil

3. Fluoxetine, because of its long plasma half-life and active metabolite, may be stopped abruptly if the dose is 20mg/day

4. If withdrawal symptoms occur (see over) slow the rate of drug withdrawal or (if drug has been stopped) give reassurance: symptoms rarely last more than 1-2 weeks. Restarting is only recommended if withdrawal is severe or prolonged.

5. When swapping from one antidepressant to another, abrupt withdrawal should usually be avoided. Cross-tapering is preferred, where the dose of the ineffective or poorly tolerated drug is slowly reduced while the new drug is slowly introduced.

Example:		**Week 1**	**Week 2**	**Week 3**	**Week 4**
Withdrawing Dothiepin	150mg OD	100mg OD	50mg OD	25mg OD	Nil
Introducing Citalopram	Nil	10mg OD	10mg OD	20mg OD	20mg OD

● The speed of cross-tapering is best judged by monitoring patient tolerability. No clear guidelines are available, so caution is required.

● Note that the co-administration of some antidepressants, even when cross-tapering, is absolutely contra-indicated. In other cases, theoretical risks or lack of experience preclude recommending cross-tapering.

● In some cases cross-tapering may not be considered necessary. An example is when switching from one SSRI to another: their effects are so similar that administration of the second drug is likely to ameliorate withdrawal effects of the first. However, there is little firm evidence of this occurring. Moreover, there are few good reasons for switching from one SSRI to another.

● Potential dangers of simultaneously administering two antidepressants include pharmacodynamic interactions (serotonin syndrome, hypotension, drowsiness) and pharmacokinetic interactions (e.g. elevation of tricyclic plasma levels by some SSRIs). See below for symptoms of serotonin syndrome.

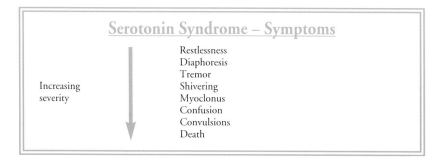

Serotonin Syndrome – Symptoms

Increasing severity

Restlessness
Diaphoresis
Tremor
Shivering
Myoclonus
Confusion
Convulsions
Death

Antidepressant discontinuation syndrome

Symptoms

Dizziness*

Electric shock sensations*

Anxiety and agitation

Insomnia

Flu-like symptoms

Diarrhoea and abdominal spasms

Paraesthesia*

Mood swings

Nausea

Low mood

* Common in SSRI/venlafaxine withdrawal

Antidepressants –

To / From	MAOIs – hydrazines	Tranyl-cypromine	Tricyclics	Citalopram	Fluoxetine	Paroxetine
MAOIs – hydrazines	Withdraw and wait for two weeks	Withdraw and wait for two weeks	Withdraw and wait for two weeks	Withdraw and wait for two weeks	Withdraw and wait for two weeks	Withdraw and wait for two weeks
Tranyl-cypromine	Withdraw and wait for two weeks	–	Withdraw and wait for two weeks	Withdraw and wait for two weeks	Withdraw and wait for two weeks	Withdraw and wait for two weeks
Tricyclics	Withdraw and wait for one week	Withdraw and wait for one week	Cross taper cautiously	Halve dose and add citalopram then slow withdrawal. [2]	Halve dose and add fluoxetine then slow withdrawal. [2]	Halve dose and add paroxetine then slow withdrawal. [2]
Citalopram	Withdraw and wait for one week	Withdraw and wait for one week	Cross taper cautiously [2]	–	Withdraw then start fluoxetine	Withdraw and start paroxetine at 10mg/day
Paroxetine	Withdraw and wait for two weeks	Withdraw and wait for one week	Cross taper cautiously with very low dose of tricyclic [2]	Withdraw and start citalopram	Withdraw then start fluoxetine	–
Fluoxetine [3]	Withdraw and wait five to six weeks	Withdraw and wait five to six weeks	Stop fluoxetine. Start tricyclic at very low dose and increase very slowly	Stop fluoxetine. Wait 4-7 days. Start citalopram at 10mg/day and increase slowly	–	Withdraw fluoxetine. Wait 4-7 days, then start paroxetine 10mg/day

– swapping and stopping

Sertraline	Trazodone/ nefazodone	Moclobemide	Reboxetine	Venlafaxine	Mirtazapine
Withdraw and wait for two weeks	Withdraw and wait for two weeks	Withdraw and wait for two weeks[*1]	Withdraw and wait for two weeks	Withdraw and wait for two weeks	Withdraw and wait for two weeks
Withdraw and wait for two weeks	Withdraw and wait for two weeks	Withdraw and wait for two weeks[*1]	Withdraw and wait for two weeks	Withdraw and wait for two weeks	Withdraw and wait for two weeks
Halve dose and add sertraline then slow withdrawal[*2]	Halve dose and add trazodone/ nefazodone, then slow withdrawal	Withdraw and wait for 1 week	Cross taper cautiously	Cross taper cautiously, starting with venlafaxine 37.5mg at night	Withdraw before starting mirtazapine cautiously
Withdraw and start sertraline at 25mg/day	Withdraw before starting titration of trazodone/ nefazodone	Withdraw and wait at least one week	Cross taper cautiously	Withdraw Start venlafaxine 37.5mg/day. Increase very slowly	Withdraw before starting mirtazapine cautiously
Withdraw and start sertraline at 25mg/day	Withdraw before starting titration of trazodone/ nefazodone	Withdraw and wait at least two weeks	Cross taper cautiously	Withdraw paroxetine. Start venlafaxine 37.5mg/day and increase very slowly	Withdraw before starting mirtazapine cautiously
Stop fluoxetine. Wait 4-7 days, then start sertraline 25mg/day	Stop fluoxetine. Wait 4-7 days then start low dose trazodone/ nefazodone	Withdraw and wait at least five weeks	Withdraw. Start reboxetine at 2mg bd and increase cautiously	Withdraw. Wait 4-7 days. Start venlafaxine at 37.5mg/day. Increase very slowly	Withdraw. Wait 4–7 days before starting mirtazapine cautiously

Antidepressants

From \ To	MAOIs – hydrazines	Tranyl-cypromine	Tricyclics	Citalopram	Fluoxetine	Paroxetine
Sertraline	Withdraw and wait for two weeks	Withdraw and wait for two weeks	Cross taper cautiously with very low dose of tricyclic. *2	Withdraw then start citalopram	Withdraw then start fluoxetine	Withdraw then start paroxetine
Trazodone/ nefazodone	Withdraw and wait at least one week.	Withdraw and wait at least one week	Cross taper cautiously with very low dose of tricyclic	Withdraw then start citalopram	Withdraw then start fluoxetine	Withdraw then start paroxetine
Moclobemide	Withdraw and wait 24 hours	Withdraw and wait 24 hours	Withdraw and wait 24 hours	Withdraw and wait 24 hours	Withdraw and wait 24 hours	Withdraw and wait 24 hours
Reboxetine	Withdraw and wait at least one week	Withdraw and wait at least one week	Cross taper cautiously	Cross taper cautiously.	Cross taper cautiously.	Cross taper cautiously.
Venlafaxine	Withdraw and wait at least one week	Withdraw and wait at least one week	Cross taper cautiously with very low dose of tricyclic *2	Cross taper cautiously. Start with 10mg/day	Cross taper cautiously. Start with 20mg every other day	Cross taper cautiously. Start with 10mg/day
Mirtazapine	Withdraw and wait for two weeks	Withdraw and wait for two weeks	Withdraw then start tricyclic	Withdraw then start citalopram	Withdraw then start fluoxetine	Withdraw then start paroxetine
Stopping *4	Reduce over four weeks	Reduce over four weeks	Reduce over four weeks	Reduce over four weeks	At 20mg/day – just stop. At 40mg/day reduce over two weeks	Reduce over four weeks or longer, if necessary *5

*1. Abrupt switching is possible but not recommended.
*2. Do not co-administer clomipramine and SSRIs or venlafaxine. Withdraw clomipramine before starting.
*3. Beware interactions with fluoxetine may still occur for five weeks after stopping fluoxetine because of long half-life.

– swapping and stopping *(Continued)*

Sertraline	Trazodone/ nefazodone	Moclobemide	Reboxetine	Venlafaxine	Mirtazapine[4]
–	Withdraw before starting trazodone/ nefazodone	Withdraw and wait at least two weeks	Cross taper cautiously	Withdraw. Start venlafaxine at 37.5mg/day	Withdraw before starting mirtazapine cautiously
Withdraw then start sertraline	–	Withdraw and wait at least one week	Withdraw, start reboxetine at 2mg BD and increase cautiously	Withdraw. Start venlafaxine at 37.5mg/day	Withdraw before starting mirtazapine cautiously
Withdraw and wait 24 hours	Withdraw and wait 24 hours	–	Withdraw and wait 24 hours	Withdraw and wait 24 hours	Withdraw and wait 24 hours
Cross taper cautiously	Cross taper cautiously	Withdraw and wait at least one week	–	Cross taper cautiously	Cross taper cautiously
Cross taper cautiously. Start with 25mg/day	Cross taper cautiously	Withdraw and wait at least one week	Cross taper cautiously	–	Withdraw before starting mirtazapine cautiously
Withdraw then start sertraline	Withdraw then start trazodone/ nefazodone	Withdraw and wait one week	Withdraw then start reboxetine	Withdraw then start venlafaxine	–
Reduce over four weeks	Reduce over four weeks	Reduce over four weeks	Reduce over four weeks	Reduce over four weeks or longer, if necessary [5]	Reduce over four weeks

*4. See general guidelines.
*5. Withdrawal effects seem to be more pronounced. Slow withdrawal over 1-3 months may be necessary.

56
ECT and Psychotropics

There have been few well-controlled studies on the use of psychotropics in ECT and much of the information available is based on clinical experience or anecdotal reports. For drugs known to lower seizure threshold it is best to start treatment with a low stimulus (50 mC). Staff should be alerted to the possibility of prolonged seizures and I/V diazepam should be available. Orientation and cognitive function should be monitored in all patients after ECT. Information contained in the table below is based on The Second Report of the Royal College of Psychiatrists' Special Committee on ECT.

Drug	Effect on ECT seizure duration	Comment
Benzodia-zepines	⬇	If possible avoid during ECT, as these will raise the seizure threshold. This includes short-acting benzos for night sedation. Those on long-term therapy should have their dosage slowly reduced and/or tapered off if clinically indicated–and if practicable–before ECT. If sedation required, consider the use of hydroxyzine.
Selective serotonin reuptake inhibitors (SSRIs)	? ⬆	Despite anecdotal reports suggesting a problem, studies indicate taking SSRIs during ECT is safe. If clinically indicated, there is no contraindication to continuing SSRIs during ECT.
Tricyclic antidepressants (TCAs)	? ⬆	No studies looking at seizure duration with TCAs during ECT but TCAs can lower seizure threshold. As some elderly patients experience asystole after ECT, it is best to avoid TCAs in elderly and those with cardiac disease. TCAs may be safely continued during ECT. Abrupt withdrawal prior to ECT is not advisable. Monitor hypotensive effects. Anticholinergic effects may predispose to confusion.
Monoamine oxidase inhibitors (MAOIs)	? –	Little information about effect on seizure threshold and few studies of use in ECT. Monitor hypotensive effects. Do not need to discontinue but _do inform anaesthetist_. No information at this time on moclobemide and ECT, although manufacturer recommends stopping it 24 hours before ECT.
Lithium	? ⬆	Literature on lithium and ECT is conflicting. One retrospective study demonstrated more cognitive problems with lithium/ECT vs ECT alone. However, two prospective studies found no such problems. Although some sources recommend stopping lithium 48 hours prior to treatment, it need not be stopped if a low stimulus is used at the start of therapy and the patient is monitored closely throughout treatment for cognitive effects and evidence of lithium toxicity.
Barbiturates	⬇	All barbiturates may shorten seizure duration and methohexital and thiopental have been reported to induce cardiac arrythmias. Nonetheless, barbiturates are frequently used for narcosis during ECT, but it is recommended that low to moderate doses be used.
Anti-psychotics	? ⬆	Few studies on antipsychotics and ECT. There are some reports of augmentation of effect when used for schizophrenia. Manufacturers recommend clozapine is suspended for 24 hours prior to ECT but safe concurrent use has been reported. Anticholinergic effects may predispose to confusion and augment effects of atropine-like pre/post-meds. May also increase risk of hypotension.
Anticon-vulsants	⬇	Continue during ECT if prescribed as mood stabiliser but may need higher energy stimulus. If used for epilepsy, their effect should be to normalise seizure threshold.

Treatment of Acute Mania / Hypomania

STEP 1

> **Start/Optimise mood-stabiliser****
> Lithium serum level 0.6 - 1.2 mmol/L*
> Carbamazepine 8 - 12 mg/L
> Valproate 50 - 100 mg/L
> Evaluate over 1-4 weeks.

If psychosis present

STEP 2

> **Begin antipsychotic**
> e.g. haloperidol   5 mg tds
> chlorpromazine   100 mg tds
> Evaluate over 2-3 weeks then discontinue slowly.

Only if ineffective

STEP 3

> **Consider other sedatives**
> e.g. lorazepam ativan   1 mg tds
> clonazepam rivotril   1 mg bd
> Discontinue after 2-4 weeks.

Only if ineffective

STEP 4

> **Consider other putative anti-manic agents**
> e.g. nimodipine; lamotrigine; Gabapentin; neurontin
> combinations of lithium/carbamazepine/valproate

---

*   Serum concentrations at higher end of therapeutic range may be required in acute mania.

**   Starting doses for mood-stabilisers:
Lithium 400mg MR OD
Carbamazepine 200mg MR BD
Valproate 500mg MR OD

Mood Stab

Name	Details	Psychiatric Indications (* Not CSM approved)	Dose
Lithium Priadel Camcolit.	Inhibits the enzyme inositol-1-phosphatase → ↑ cellular responses linked to PI 2nd messenger system 1/2 life: 20hrs Renal excretion, no metabolism	Acute mania, Prophylaxis of bipolar disorder, Adjunctive treatment in resistant depression, Schizoaffective disorder, Violent patients (also with mental handicap)	Start on low (400 mg) dose; Serum concs to be monitored every 5 to 7 days until level is between 0.6 – 1.0mmol/L Thereafter check levels every 2-3 months NB. all samples must be taken 12 hours post dose
Carbamazepine TEGRETOL	Possible peripheral benzodiazepine receptor agonist (located on GABA$_A$ receptor complex). GABA principal inhibitory peptide in brain. Peripheral benzodiazepine receptor regulates Ca^{++} channel function. ? Stops kindling process 1/2 life: 12-17 hours Metabolised by liver & then excreted by kidney retarding electrical discharges in the limbic system.	Prophylaxis of bipolar illness * Rapid Cycling. (both indications- alone or in combination with Li$^+$) * Acute mania ▲ Anti-convulsant. Use if patient is unresponsive to Li.	Usual starting-dose 200mg BD, slowly increased until dose 600-1,000mg/ day is achieved. MR prep possibly better tolerated Target range for psychiatric: 8-12 mg/l Sample at trough Induces own metabolism: monitor every two weeks until stable then every 3-6 months

ilising Agents

Precautions	Contraindications	Side Effects	Drug Interactions
1. Renal function: U&E before commencing Li⁺. Excreted through kidney exclusively: potentially nephrotoxic. Change in body salt concentration can affect levels 2. 3-4% develop hypothyroidism: TFT before starting & six-monthly intervals. 3. Lithium toxicity > levels 1.5mmol/L 4. Baseline ECG Should get Li⁺ card from pharmacy.	Pregnancy – consult Drug Information Service Breast-feeding – avoid Renal impairment (may be given if close monitoring practicable) Thyroidopathies Sick Sinus Syndrome	Thirst, polyuria GI upset Tremor (may treat with propranolol) Diabetes insipidus – may inhibit ADH (must maintain fluid intake) Acne Muscular weakness Cardiac arrhythmias Weight gain common (? related to thirst & intake of high calorie drinks) Hypothyroidism	**Antipsychotics** – all antipsychotics may increase lithium's neurotoxicity **Diuretics** (thiazides): increase Li⁺ concentration **ACE inhibitors**: toxicity **Diltiazem/Verapamil:** neurotoxicity **Xanthines**: increase Li⁺ excretion **NaCl**: increases Li⁺ excretion **Alcohol**: increases peak Li⁺ concentration **NSAIDs**: all cause toxicity except aspirin & sulindac. Low dose ibuprofen usually safe. → non steroidal Anti-Inflammitory drugs.
1. Warn about fever, infections etc: Need pre + regular FBCs every 2 weeks for 1st 2 months. Early leucopenias usually transient and benign. 2. Carbamazepine toxicity: diplopia, ataxia, sedation	Pregnancy – consult Drug Information Service Breast-feeding Possibly alcohol abuse, glaucoma, diabetes	jerky movements ① Drowsiness, ataxia, double vision diplopia, nausea Agranulocytosis – 1 in 20,000 Aplastic anaemia – 1 in 20,000 Transient leucopenias in approx. 10% in 1st 2 months Hypersensitivity-hepatitis Rashes SIADH	**Antipsychotics:** may cause CNS effects (drowsiness, ataxia etc.) **Lithium:** CNS effects and increased risk of side effects of both drugs **Ca⁺⁺ channel blockers**: CNS effects **MAOIs:** Need 2 weeks washout ↓ **TCA/ neuroleptic** ?Toxicity with 'Flu Vaccine Enzyme inducer: affects many others including **phenytoin** and oral contraceptives.

Mood Stab

Name	Details	Psychiatric Indications (* Not CSM approved)	Dose
Sodium Valproate EPILIM	↓ catabolism of g - aminobutyric acid 1/2 life of 8 hours Metabolised **Membrane Stabilising** activity.	In cases of failure with lithium or carbamazepine: *Acute mania – especially mixed affective states * Prophylaxis of manic and depressive episodes ★ Anti- convulsants.	Commence on 500mg MR daily. Then increase until plasma levels reach 50-100mg/l Trough samples required M/R prep may be given once daily
Clonazepam RIVOTRIL	Rapidly Absorbed: No major metabolites 1/2 life: 34 hours	* Acute mania * Adjunctive therapy with lithium in prophylaxis of bipolar disorder	1mg initially at night, ↑to 4-8mg/day over 4 weeks (divided doses)
Verapamil (Nimodipine)	Ca⁺⁺ channel blocker-inhibits Ca⁺⁺ dependent intra-cellular protein kinases 1/2 life: 5-12 hours	In cases of failure with lithium or carbamazepine:- * Acute mania * Prophylaxis of bipolar disorder * Rapid cycling	40mg TDS initially, up to 80-120mg TDS (slow increase). M/R preps may aid compliance Nimodipine – 60mg tds
Lamotrigine	1/2 life: 20-24 hours but 1/2 life increased by valproate and decreased by enzyme inducers	In cases of failure with lithium, carbamazepine or valproate * Acute mania * Prophylaxis of bipolar disorder * Rapid cycling	Dose as mood stabilizer not certain, likely similar to that used in epilepsy. As dose depends on concomitant medication, see Manufacturer's information.

ilising Agents

Precautions	Contraindications	Possible Side Effects	Drug Interactions
1. Check renal & hepatic function regularly (including baseline) 2. FBC regularly	Pregnancy – consult Drug Information Service Breast-feeding Hepatic disease	Commonly: Nausea, vomiting, Sedation Rarely: Ataxia, Headache, Anxiety, Thrombocytopenia & platelet dysfunction Pancreatitis	Complex interactions with other anticonvulsants: need to consult neurologist or Drug Information Potentiates activity of aspirin & warfarin May increase MAOI & TCA levels
1. Check hepatic & renal function regularly 2. FBC regularly 3. Avoid sudden withdrawal	Respiratory depression Porphyria	Commonly: Drowsiness, Fatigue, Dizziness, Muscle Hypotonia	Ataxia & dysarthria possibly with lithium or antipsychotics Additive CNS depressant effects Increased levels of phenytoin
1. Monitor BP, pulse 2. Monitor ECG 3. Elderly	Conduction defects (myocardial) Pregnancy Breast-feeding Cardiac failure	Hypotension, Bradycardia, AV block, G I Symptoms – constipation very common with verapamil, rare with nimodipine	Neurotoxicity with lithium or carbamazepine Other hypotensives Antiarrhythmics Digoxin Beta-blockers – can be fatal with verapamil
1. Monitor patient for rash – more likely to occur in children, with concomitant valproate or if dose started too high or increased too quickly. Most rashes occur within 8 weeks of starting therapy.	Pregnancy – consult Drug Information Service Hepatic impairment	Rash, Ataxia, Diplopia, Headache, Vomiting	Valproate increases levels of lamotrigine Lamotrigine may increase levels of the carbamazepine epoxide metabolite

Algorithm for the Treatment of Rapid-Cycling Bipolar Affective Disorder

1st Line	or	Lithium
	or	Carbamazepine
		Valproate
2nd Line		Combine two or more first line drugs
3rd Line		Add thyroxine *(to double free thyroid levels)*
4th Line		Withdraw thyroxine
		Add Nimodipine *(30-60mg tds)*
5th Line		Withdraw Nimodipine
		Add Clozapine

Notes

* Rapid cycling = more than four episodes of (hypo)mania/depression in a 12 month period
* Take a detailed history and consider precipitants of mood change which might be predicted or controlled (eg external stressors, life events and changes during menstrual cycle).
* Target plasma levels (at trough) are:

  Lithium   0.6 - 1.0 mmol/l
  Carbamazepine   8 -12 mg/l
  Valproate   50-100 mg/l

* Clozapine is not licensed for use in bipolar disorder. Do not use with carbamazepine.
* Other neuroleptics may be used but should usually be reserved for 'when necessary' treatment of hypomanic symptoms. Continuous therapy is not recommended because of long term adverse effects such as tardive dyskinesia.
* Lamotrigine may be effective but few data at present.

IV

Treatment of
Anxiety

Use of Anxiolytics and Hypnotics

I) Anxiolytics

Anxiety or concern about circumstances in life is common and not necessarily pathological. A range of disorders come under the heading of Anxiety Disorders, the most common being that of generalised anxiety disorder (GAD) with a prevalence of around 3%. Physical causes of anxiety must be excluded (e.g. thyroid disorder; drug/caffeine abuse). Anxiety disorders often occur with other psychiatric disorders, particularly depression.

Treatment of Anxiety Disorders

Disorder	Behavioural/ Nonpharmacological Therapies	Recommended Psychotropics
Generalised Anxiety Disorder	Relaxation; Biofeedback; Cognitive therapy; Anxiety management; Psychotherapy	Propranolol (for prominant somatic symptoms) Avoid short-acting benzodiazepines; (Consider diazepam) Buspirone ? Paroxetine ? Venlafaxine
Simple Phobia	Exposure in vivo; Systematic desensitization	None
Social Phobia	Anxiety management	Paroxetine, Propranolol, MAOIs
Obsessive-Compulsive Disorder	Thought stopping; Exposure in vivo; Response prevention	Fluoxetine, Paroxetine, Clomipramine
Panic Disorder	Cognitive therapy; Anxiety management	Citalopram Paroxetine, MAOIs, Diazepam, Imipramine

◆ *Benzodiazepines* - longer acting compounds such as diazepam are preferred in short-term use and for withdrawal regimes. Oxazepam is a metabolite of diazepam and is shorter acting. Lorazepam is often used parenterally for acute agitation in psychosis, but should be avoided in anxious patients. Marked tolerance and withdrawal phenomena can occur.

◆ *Buspirone* - 5HT1a receptor agonist; effect is generally thought to be small, especially in benzodiazepine users; slow onset (up to 4 weeks); no interaction with alcohol or other psychotropics; minimal tolerance and withdrawal.

◆ *Beta-blockers* - used in situational anxiety especially for prominent somatic symptoms; safe with no withdrawal or dependence potential; may cause side-effects (e.g. drowsiness, nightmares and low mood in chronic use) or interact with other drugs.

◆ *Antidepressants* - the SSRIs, fluoxetine, paroxetine and sertraline, are all licensed for anxiety associated with depression. Trazodone has anxiolytic activity and is relatively safe. Imipramine and clomipramine may also be effective, particularly for panic disorder and for obsessive-compulsive disorder. Evidence is emerging that venlafaxine may be effective in GAD. Phenelzine and moclobemide may also be effective in phobias.

II) Hypnotics

Before treating insomnia with drugs:

Take a thorough sleep history

Is the insomnia initial or middle insomnia? Is there early morning wakening? Consider whole lifetime: most 1° insomniacs have always been poor sleepers.

Determine the pattern of sleep

Is the sleep pattern normal? Has the diurnal rhythm become disturbed? Are other factors (nightwork; jet-lag) involved?

Duration of disturbance

Is the sleep disturbance chronic and stable or acute?

Look for possible causes of sleep disturbance

✧ Psychiatric illness e.g. anxiety disorder, depression, acute psychosis, mania.

✧ Drug-induced (theophylline, sympathomimetics, caffeine, nocturnal anticholinergics, tranylcypromine, etc).

✧ Drug-withdrawal in dependence (consider affect of withdrawal from therapeutic agents).

✧ Medical disorder e.g. thyroid disease, menopausal symptoms, peptic ulceration due to excessive alcohol or caffeine, any pain.

✧ Coming into hospital or other change of environment.

Think about alternative treatments

Sleep hygiene:

✦ Avoid daytime naps/resting/reading in bed; reduce caffeine intake; anxiety management; relaxation techniques. Encourage patient to go to bed at same time; reserve bed for sleep.

✦ Always treat underlying causes.

If hypnotics are to be prescribed:

❖ With nursing staff, counsel patient about the use of hypnotics: explain that they may only be used for a short time. Outline risks of tolerance, dependence and withdrawal.

General guidelines on hypnotic use:

❖ Avoid short-acting, high potency benzodiazepines e.g. lorazepam. Oxazepam is preferable. Note abuse potential of temazepam.

❖ Alternative compounds include antihistamines (e.g. promethazine), zopiclone and zolpidem.

❖ Avoid high doses.

❖ Short-term use only (no more than 2 weeks) with regular review; intermittent if possible.

❖ Avoid abrupt withdrawal, if use has been continuous for <2 weeks.

❖ Avoid in respiratory failure and in addiction-prone individuals.

❖ Reduce doses in the elderly.

❖ Note all antihistamines are long-acting with noticeable hangover. Some have slow onset of effect.

Benzodiazepine Oral Dose Equivalents

Benzodiazepine	Equivalent Diazepam Dose	Approximate Duration of Action
Diazepam	5mg	2-4 days
Chlordiazepoxide	15mg (10-25mg)	2-4 days
Clonazepam	0.5mg (0.25-2mg)	1-2 days
Lorazepam	0.5 (0.5-1mg)	8-12 hours
Nitrazepam	5mg (2.5-10mg)	12-24 hours
Oxazepam	15mg (5-30mg)	8-12 hours
Temazepam	10mg (7.5-15mg)	8 hours

Benzodiazepine Oral / Parenteral Dose Equivalents

Drug	Oral Dose	Equivalent IV or IM dose (mg)
Diazepam	10	10
Lorazepam	4	4

V

Treatment of
Special Patient Populations

Treatment of Childhood Psychiatric Illness

Hyperkinetic Disorder

Children who meet the ICD-10 criteria for hyperkinetic disorder (HD) should have a treatment plan that includes the reduction of hyperactive behaviour as one of the goals. It is not the only goal: it will also be important to detect and treat any coexisting disorders, to prevent the development of conduct disorder (or reduce it if it has developed), to promote academic and social learning, improve emotional adjustment and self-esteem and relieve family distress. A multimodal treatment approach will usually be needed.

Medication

Initial medication should be as a trial. Placebo control is not routinely necessary but helps in problem cases. Medication should be discussed and explained with the child, parents and teachers before it is started. While medication is being started, the family will need quick and ready access to the prescriber to report progress and any adverse effects.

Methylphenidate and dexamphetamine are the only drugs licensed in the UK for the treatment of hyperactivity. The use of non-licensed drugs, or polypharmacy, should be on the advice of a specialist. Both stimulants have broadly similar effects on children's behaviour: they reduce hyperactive behaviour, enhance several aspects of information processing and increase on-task attentiveness.

Drug Choice

Methylphenidate will usually be the first choice, but dexamphetamine may be preferred if the child has epilepsy. Pemoline has been used in the past but is now withdrawn from the market because of toxicity and is available only on a named patient basis in the UK.

Dose

The starting dose of methylphenidate is 5.0 mg (dexamphetamine 2.5 mg) twice daily with the dose being adjusted in the light of response. The dose may need to rise as high as 15mg three times daily. If a dose range higher than that is contemplated, then more intensive monitoring should be used and a specialist consulted. Several doses a day are usually needed. Psychological action has a peak in the first hour and the effect wanes rapidly, with little action after about four hours. Accordingly, most children will be losing the effect of a breakfast dose by midday. Subsequent doses may then have to be given at school. Methylphenidate slow release tablets are available in some countries and can be imported to the UK.

Evaluation

Psychological response should be monitored with rating scales of behaviours (e.g. Conners abbreviated scale) completed regularly and systematically in different settings - e.g. by parents and school. Re-evaluation at the clinic should be carried out when rating scales suggest that a therapeutic response is being achieved, or if there is no response after a month of therapy. Physical monitoring should include the plotting of height and weight along standardised growth curves, and examination for the appearance of any tics. Adverse psychological effects such as lack of spontaneity, depression and excessive perseveration should be assessed specifically, with ratings, interview and observation methods. Questioning should elicit any difficulties in getting to sleep, appetite disturbances, stomach-aches, headaches and dizziness. Many of the adverse effects of stimulants are transient and decrease with time.

The aim is to maintain medication until the child's maturation and learning of cognitive skills make medication unnecessary. Periodically, approximately annually, there should be a gradual withdrawal of medication over a period of two weeks to assess whether there is indeed a continuing need for medication. Drug holidays - e.g. during weekends and vacations from school - are not required routinely unless the child's growth has been affected by medication.

Attention Deficit/Hyperactivity Disorder

These suggestions for medication have been developed for the treatment of hyperkinetic disorder. For children with lesser degrees of hyperactivity - i.e. those with a DSM-IV diagnosis of Attention Deficit/Hyperactivity (ADHD), but not HD - underlying causes such as learning disabilities, hearing impairment, family stresses, attachment disruptions and emotional disorders, should be carefully sought. Indications for medication in this group will usually arise only if the problems have not resolved with approaches designed to remove environmental causes or treat psychologically. There may be a temptation to rely unduly on the effect of medication and to use for mild cases where educational intervention and psychological treatment would be sufficient.

Unlicensed drugs

Antidepressants

Stimulants will fail to produce a clinically significant change in behaviour in about 10% to 30% of treated children. In them, and in children with tics or mood disorders, a tricyclic antidepressant can be a useful alternative. The dose (approx. 1 mg imipramine/kg body weight) is less than that for treating depression and the onset is quicker, usually in the first 3 days of treatment. The serious hazards are for the cardiovascular system: there can be tachycardia and deterioration of the ECG even two years after the start of the treatment. A few cases with sudden death, presumably due to cardiac arrhythmia, have been reported in children using desipramine. Repeated ECGs and blood estimations (monthly at the start of treatment, quarterly after 6 months) are needed with doses over 50 mg daily of imipramine. Warning signs include a P-R interval more than 200 msec., a QRS interval more than 120 msec., or a serum level of imipramine and its metabolite desipramine above 300 ng/ml. Female patients seem to reach higher blood levels with the same weight-adjusted dose than male patients, and also show more side-effects. The blood level is markedly and unpredictably increased if methylphenidate is given simultaneously, so the combination should be given, if at all, only with close monitoring of blood level and ECG. In adolescents suicidal behaviour is increasing, so special care is needed and a good relationship between physician, parents and child is required.

Clonidine

Clonidine (50 to 100 mcg daily in two divided doses) has some effect in reducing hyperactive behaviour, though little benefit on cognitive performance can be expected. It does not worsen tics, and may even improve them.

Low-dose haloperidol reduces hyperactivity through a different mechanism from the stimulants and may be effective when they fail; but dystonias can appear in children even at these very low doses so it should be regarded as a treatment of last resort. Risperidone has not undergone formal trials but is a safe alternative, although EPS can occur. New and promising drugs such as moclobemide are still under evaluation.

Younger Children

Methylphenidate is officially not recommended below the age of 6, though it is hard to see why the manufacturers have taken this line given the scientific evidence. Dexamphetamine is licensed down to the age of 3 years. Clinicians should diagnose and treat hyperkinetic disorders from the age of 4 years, but should do so with some caution, remembering the difficulties of diagnosis in this age group and the possibility that oppositional and noncompliant behaviour may be mislabelled as Attention Deficit.

Depression in Children

Depression is now felt to occur more commonly in children than previously thought. Symptoms may be more varied in children than in adults and comorbidity, particularly with anxiety disorders, is common. In contrast to adult studies, controlled trials of tricyclic antidepressants in children have not shown consistent efficacy over placebo. In view of this lack of effect and their known hazards, TCAs should be prescribed only after specialist consultation and with ECG monitoring (see above). SSRIs should be considered the antidepressant treatment of choice in children since there is preliminary trial evidence of efficacy and they have fewer cardiac and anticholinergic side effects and are less sedating. This in spite of the manufacturers' statement that they are not recommended in childhood. Treatment with SSRIs is much easier to monitor, the drugs are far better tolerated and are safer in overdose. As there are no studies to recommend any one SSRI, adherence and tolerability are the main factors in the choice of drug. If adherence is a likely problem, fluoxetine may be the preferred SSRI as the child or adolescent is much less likely to suffer from a discontinuation syndrome with intermittent usage. Fluoxetine and paroxetine are also available as a liquid preparation which can be advantageous in this population. The prescription and monitoring of SSRIs in children are similar to adults. Augmentation strategies can also be tried but this should only occur after specialist consultation. Depression in children should always be looked at in the full context in which it occurs and family, school and environmental factors considered. Cognitive behavioural therapy, interpersonal psychotherapy, counseling and other non-pharmacological approaches are all useful in this population.

Psychosis in Children

Schizophrenia is rare in children but increases markedly in incidence in adolescence. Early onset schizophrenia (EOS) is generally considered to be a variant of the adult form of schizophrenia. From a treatment perspective, it is best to conceptualise EOS as such, despite the differences from adult forms (eg outcomes, neurodevelopmental abnormalities, familial risk, and premorbid personality factors). It is often difficult to differentiate schizophrenia from bipolar mood disorder associated with psychosis in children. Careful follow-up of children presenting with psychosis is thus necessary in order to monitor the long-term course of the illness. Both schizophrenia and bipolar disorder with psychosis have a devastating effect on academic and social development.

There is a paucity of research into the use of antipsychotics in children. What research there is increasingly indicates pharmacotherapy is effective. Children are more susceptible to EPS and this may affect choice of antipsychotic. Hyperprolactinaemia and weight gain are also important considerations in antipsychotic choice in this population. Genetics, neurodevelopmental factors, family and school dynamics and other issues in management of psychiatric illness in children mean that one must take a multidisciplinary approach to treatment in this population and include the family, teachers, social workers, pharmacist, paediatrician and GP in the treatment plan.

Psychotropic Group	Recommended drugs
Drugs for Treatment of Hyperkinetic Disorder	Methylphenidate Dexamphetamine (See above) Other treatment options (See above): TCAs e.g. 1mg/kg imipramine/day Clonidine 50 - 100mcg/day Haloperidol* 0.02 – 0.08mg/kg/day
Antipsychotics*	Risperidone 2 - 4mg/day Olanzapine 2.5 - 15mg/day Clozapine up to 5 mg/kg (start with 12.5 mg/day)
Antidepressants	Fluoxetine 10 - 20mg/day Paroxetine 10 - 40mg/day Sertraline 25 – 100mg/day
Drugs for Treatment of Nocturnal Enuresis	Desmopressin 20 - 40 mcg nocte intranasally Imipramine 0.5 - 1.5 mg/kg

*(Dystonias/dyskinesias very common in children; consider making procyclidine available to family)

The Elderly

General rules

❖　　The elderly have an *increased sensitivity to medications* as a result of age-related alterations in pharmacodynamics (changes in neuronal cell numbers, receptors and receptor binding) and pharmacokinetics (changes in absorption, distribution, metabolism, excretion and protein binding).

❖　　*Changes in hepatic metabolism* include a decrease in the first pass effects, as well as a decrease in oxidation, reduction and hydrolysis (phase I enzymatic reactions) of drugs. Drugs metabolised by first pass effects will thus have an increased bioavailability. Lipophilic drugs will demonstrate an increased apparent volume of distribution, while this will be decreased for hydrophilic agents. Drugs with an increased volume of distribution and a decreased hepatic clearance (e.g. diazepam) and those requiring oxidation for biotransformation will thus have a greatly prolonged half-life. *Renal clearance* declines gradually with age and this may affect clearance of many drugs (see McConnell and Duffy, 1994).

❖　　As a result of this increased sensitivity, the lowest effective dosage of medications should be used: i.e. *start low, go slow, monitor effects frequently.*

❖　　Always identify possible determinants of medication *noncompliance,* including social (e.g. living alone, financial situation), physical (e.g. hearing and visual loss), concomitant illness and cognitive factors.

❖　　Consider the possibility of concomitant use of *over the counter (OTC) medications.*

❖　　Always *consider drug toxicity* when the patient exhibits alterations in attention or cognition or any behavioural change.

❖　　*Avoid polypharmacy;* the elderly are at increased risk of adverse neuropsychiatric complications from drug interactions.

❖　　Highly *protein bound drugs* will have increased free plasma levels if albumin levels are reduced. This may not be reflected in routine laboratory testing of total drug concentrations only.

❖　　Avoid the use of drugs which put the elderly at *risk for falls*, especially sedative-hypnotics, phenobarbitone, phenytoin.

❖　　Consider the use of psychotherapy and other *nonpharmacological treatments.*

Choice of psychotropics

❖　　The elderly are more sensitive to orthostatic hypotension and anticholinergic effects. *Tricyclics* should be used with caution and monoamine oxidase inhibitors (MAOIs) should be avoided. *SSRIs* and *moclobemide* may be better tolerated and have fewer cardiac effects. Of the SSRIs, the half-lives of sertraline and citalopram are prolonged in the elderly. If a tricyclic antidepressant is required, nortriptyline may be better tolerated. Amoxapine should be avoided because of its potential for causing EPS in this at risk population, as should tricyclics with a greater degree of anticholinergic activity. Trazodone and nefazodone may also be antidepressants of choice because they have fewer cardiac and anticholinergic effects. Orthostatic hypotension may need to be monitored, however. MAOIs should be avoided because of their propensity to cause orthostatic hypotension and because the dietary restrictions may be difficult to follow for some.

❖ *Electroconvulsive therapy (ECT)* is a safe and effective treatment option in this population for severe depression and for mania and may be better tolerated than pharmacotherapy in some patients.

❖ For late-onset *bipolar disorder*, lithium appears to be as effective as in early-onset cases, but long-term follow-up studies have not been done to date. Lithium toxicity may occur at levels that would be considered 'therapeutic' in younger patients. Lithium clearance is reduced in the elderly and doses may be up to 50% lower. Of AED mood stabilisers, carbamazepine has more adverse cardiac effects and needs to be monitored with ECGs in the elderly and sodium valproate may thus be preferred. The half-life of valproate may be longer in the elderly and the free fraction may also be increased (see Snyder and McConnell, 1998).

❖ The elderly are much more susceptible to the extrapyramidal symptoms (EPS) of *antipsychotics* as well as to the orthostatic hypotension and anticholinergic effects of these agents. When indicated they should be used in much lower doses (generally one half to one third of doses in younger adults) and titrated more slowly with frequent monitoring. It is useful to monitor the elderly for Parkinsonian side effects and for tardive dyskinesia on a three monthly basis and more frequently at the onset of therapy or when making dose adjustments. Clozapine may be associated with an increased incidence of agranulocytosis in the elderly and anecdotally has not been thought as effective as in younger adults. Sertindole should not be used in the elderly because of its cardiac effects and drug interactions. Risperidone may be used in the elderly, but its half life may be increased and blood pressure should be monitored. The lesser cardiac, anticholinergic and extrapyramidal effects of sulpiride and olanzapine make these drugs of choice in this population.

❖ *Benzodiazepines* and *drugs with a high degree of anticholinergic activity* should be avoided.

Psychotropic classification	Recommended drugs
Antidepressants	Moclobemide SSRIs
Antipsychotics	Olanzapine Risperidone Sulpiride
Mood stabilisers	Lithium Sodium Valproate

Pregnancy and Lactation

Pregnancy

Preconception

● For patients who are planning a pregnancy, discuss the risks and benefits of slowly withdrawing their medication; these will depend on the patient's history and the drugs being taken.

● Approximately 50% of pregnancies in the UK are unplanned. In view of this, when first prescribing for any woman of child-bearing age, it is important to consider the 'risk' of pregnancy and the possible effects for the foetus. For example, drugs such as lithium should not be prescribed to women of childbearing age without a prior negative pregnancy test and a discussion with the patient about the risks should she conceive.

● Women who are taking psychotropic medication and are having problems conceiving should be given a trial off medication, if clinically appropriate. Even if there is no history of menstrual cycle irregularity and investigations such as plasma prolactin levels are all normal, there may be non-specific effects on the hypothalamic-gonadotrophin axis which may hamper conception, e.g. reduced libido.

● If possible avoid all drugs especially in the first trimester. For patients who are planning a pregnancy, consider withdrawing slowly their medication (depending on the nature and severity of the patient's illness). Women may be anxious about potential harm to the foetus but the risk of relapse must be considered. Individualised counselling is advised.

● In women maintained on agents on which there are limited data, it may be appropriate to consider switching to a recommended treatment before conception. If doubt exists as to the safety of the patient's regime in pregnancy, the clinician is advised to contact their local or national drug information service.

Pregnancy

○ Always treat with the lowest effective dose, for the shortest time and review regularly. Progress should ideally be monitored using recognised rating scales such as BPRS, MADRS and HAM-D. This is especially important in busy clinics where patients may see more than one doctor.

○ In most circumstances the patient who becomes pregnant while receiving effective treatment for a psychiatric disorder should remain on the treatment known to be effective for that individual.

○ There are few data on relapse rates in pregnancy in women with a history of depression who stop their medication. Relapse may increase the risk of postpartum depression as well as cause inadequate prenatal care, poor nutrition and obstetric complications. The woman's previous psychiatric history including severity and course of illness must be taken into account when considering stopping medication. Few data exist on relapse rates in pregnant women with bipolar affective disorder who discontinue mood stabilisers.

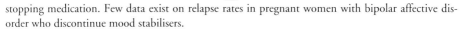 Maintaining a pregnant woman on prophylactic antipsychotic medication may be preferable to risking relapse (when higher doses of drugs may be required). Maternal relapse may also have other adverse effects on the foetus.

Ο The expected incidence of major malformations is 2 to 3% at birth with the incidence increasing to 5% by 4-5 years of age. (The incidence increases because at birth only major malformations are noted whereas by 4-5 years of age other problems such as learning difficulties and motor neurone effects are picked up.) Of these, approximately 20 to 25% will be of genetic origin, 65 to 70% will be of unknown aetiology and 1 to 3% will be caused by drugs. The expected incidence of minor anomalies is 10% and of spontaneous abortions (in clinically recognised pregnancies) 10–20%.

Ο The time of maximum teratogenic potential is approximately 17 – 60 days after conception, although developmental problems may still occur in the second and third trimesters.

Ο Synergy can occur among teratogenic agents. For instance, in one study it was noted that with antiepileptic medication, the incidence of major malformations with one drug was 4% whereas this increased to 23% with four AEDs. Ideally therefore women should be maintained on monotherapy.

Ο Try to avoid drugs that are hypotensive or anticholinergic. These effects may compound problems already seen in the patient eg: constipation. Sedative drugs may also worsen the fatigue experienced in pregnancy.

Ο Pharmacokinetics change during pregnancy and doses may need to be adjusted. For instance, volume of distribution increases, albumin levels decrease (and thus free levels of certain drugs e.g. phenytoin will need to be monitored), renal plasma flow increases and some liver metabolic pathways are induced resulting in lower plasma levels of some drugs. Because of this, plasma level monitoring of psychotropics should be undertaken if possible. For lithium and perhaps TCAs the dose will need to be increased. It is less certain for other drugs. See individual sections.

Ο As withdrawal effects (irritability, restlessness, irritability, continual crying, hypertonia, tachycardia and seizures) can occur in the newborn, psychotropics should be gradually withdrawn, if possible, during the three to four weeks before expected delivery. As this is not often practical, the newborn will need to be monitored closely for adverse effects.

Postpartum mood disorders

◆ Postpartum mood disorders include postpartum blues, nonpsychotic postpartum depression and puerperal psychosis (a form of affective psychosis related to bipolar disorder).

◆ Postpartum blues occurs in up to 75% of women. Symptoms such as a labile mood, tearfulness, generalised anxiety and sleep and appetite disturbance begin within a few days of delivery and typically remit by the tenth postpartum day. Drug treatment is not necessary.

◆ Postpartum depression occurs in 10 to 15% of women after childbirth and symptoms are similar to a nonpuerperal depression. Supportive counselling may be all that is required in most cases but approximately one-quarter of postpartum depressions will require treatment.

◆ Postpartum depression typically begins in the first two to six weeks after delivery but may occur later on. The Edinburgh Postnatal Depression Scale (EPDS) can be used to screen for the disorder.

◆ Postpartum depression occurs in 25% to 50% of women with a previous episode of postpartum depression and in 30% of women with a previous history of major depression. Sub-clinical depressive or anxiety symptoms during pregnancy can also increase the risk, as may social factors such as marital problems, poor support, adverse life events and social problems.

◆ Prophylactic antidepressant treatment has been shown to reduce relapse rates if given immediately after delivery. If postpartum depression does occur, women should be treated as if they have a nonpuerperal depressive illness and be given an adequate dose of antidepressant (eg. 150mg amitriptyline) for an adequate period i.e. six months. Antidepressants that have been investigated in postpartum depression include sertraline, venlafaxine, fluoxetine as well as oestrogen and progesterone. Antidepressant choice should however be based on previous response and the adverse effect profile of the antidepressant. When deciding whether or not to treat prescribers must be aware that maternal depression may have long-term adverse effects on the psychological development of the child. This is particularly the case if the depression occurs in the first year of life.

◆ Postpartum psychosis occurs in approximately 0.1% to 0.2% (1 to 2 per 1000) of women postpartum and presents generally within the first two weeks after delivery. Symptoms include restlessness, irritability, sleep disturbance, mood lability, disorganised behaviour, delusions and hallucinations. In women with a history of postpartum psychosis the risk of developing the illness again postpartum is 30% to 50%.

◆ In women with a history of bipolar disorder, relapse rates of 30% to 50% are seen after subsequent deliveries. The maximum risk period is in the first two years after an episode of bipolar disorder. Manic symptoms are most likely to occur in the two weeks after delivery and have a more acute onset than mania occurring outside the puerperium. Because of these high relapse rates, prophylactic lithium therapy has been investigated and found to be useful if started 48 hours postpartum in women with bipolar disorder or puerperal psychosis. Oestrogen therapy is also currently being tried and preliminary results are encouraging.

◆ *For more information on mood disorders in the postpartum period see Marks and Kumar (1998) and Kendell at al. (1987).*

Drug Choice in Pregnancy

✳   There has been limited investigation of the safety of most antipsychotics and antidepressants and conflicting data published. However, there is no good evidence to support an association between these agents and an increased risk of birth defects. Drugs with which there has been the most experience are generally regarded as being the preferred option.

✳   In depression, *tricyclic antidepressants (TCAs)* are the agents of choice as there is most experience with their use. Of these there is most experience with *amitriptyline* and *imipramine*. As these drugs are sedating, cause anticholinergic effects and postural hypotension, some suggest the use of *nortriptyline* or *desipramine* (discontinued and now only available on a named-patient basis in the UK). As dose adjustments are sometimes required in pregnancy, some suggest plasma levels of antidepressants be taken before pregnancy and once each trimester. Others however recommend that they are taken before or early on in pregnancy and then if depression recurs during pregnancy, plasma levels can again be retaken and the dose adjusted according to the plasma level. For TCAs the dose may need to be increased during pregnancy with a corresponding reduction to pregravid levels by one month postpartum.

✳   In certain circumstances *SSRIs* may be appropriate but there are fewer data on their use. There are most data for *fluoxetine* which is not thought to be associated with obstetric complications or foetal malformations. Data are encouraging with *fluvoxamine*, *paroxetine* and *sertraline* but are still too limited to recommend their use in pregnancy.

✳   Long term effects of these agents, particularly on cognitive and language functions, are even less certain. In one study, global IQ and language development were assessed in the children of mothers taking tricyclic antidepressants (n=80) or fluoxetine (n=55) during pregnancy and in a control group (n=84). The children were evaluated between the ages of 16 and 86 months and no significant differences between the groups were found. This needs replicating.

✳   *MAOIs* should be avoided as they are known to be teratogenic in animals and there are few data available on their use in pregnancy or on pregnancy outcome.

✳   There are few data on *moclobemide, venlafaxine, nefazodone, reboxetine* and *mirtazapine* and these drugs should be avoided in pregnancy.

✳   Of the *antipsychotics*, there are most data on *chlorpromazine* and *trifluoperazine* and so many consider these to be the agents of choice. Others think that low-potency agents (e.g. chlorpromazine) be avoided because they have the potential to lower blood pressure and they are anticholinergic and sedating. However, this needs to be weighed up against the risk of EPS being more likely to occur with high-potency drugs that would then require treatment with anticholinergic medication. Where data does exist for antipsychotics it generally concerns their use as antiemetics where lower doses were used for short periods. Studies on the offspring of mothers treated with phenothiazines during pregnancy have failed to show an adverse effect on cognitive function in early childhood.

✳   *Depot antipsychotics* are best avoided (if avoidance is not precluded by poor maternal adherence) as they may complicate drug withdrawal before the estimated delivery date. Neonatal withdrawal may also be more severe if depot preparations are used near term.

*   There are few data on the use of *anticholinergics* in pregnancy or on pregnancy outcome. *Benztropine* and *benzhexol* use in pregnancy may be associated with malformations although data are limited. *Diphenhydramine* (predominantly used in The USA as an anticholinergic) is considered to be safe by some although withdrawal effects in the newborn (tremulousness and diarrhoea) may occur. Other obvious effects include worsening constipation in the pregnant woman. Because there are few data with these agents, they should not be given routinely as prophylaxis during pregnancy. If EPS occur, some consider it best to switch to a low-potency antipsychotic that would be less likely to cause EPS. As with other psychotropic medication, gradual withdrawal three to four weeks before expected delivery should occur, if possible.

*   Of the mood stabilisers, *lithium, carbamazepine* and *sodium valproate* are all teratogenic and should be avoided in the first trimester, if possible. *Lithium* use is associated with Ebstein's anomaly, which is likely to occur 10 – 20 times more frequently in the infants of women exposed to lithium in the first trimester. However, as the baseline risk for Ebstein's anomaly is 1 in 20,000, the absolute risk is only 1 in 1000 or 0.1%. This is much lower than originally thought. Nevertheless, a detailed ultrasound and foetal echocardiogram should be performed at 16 to 18 weeks to rule out cardiovascular anomalies.

The risk of abnormalities occurring must be weighed against the risk of relapse in the woman if therapy is withdrawn. Relapse rates of up to 50% have been found to occur within two to ten weeks of stopping lithium therapy in patients with bipolar disorder who were treated for an average of 30 months. The risk of relapse increases with the number of prior affective episodes, poor recovery between episodes, polytherapy and if rapid discontinuation (<2 weeks) occurs. Although some have advocated rapid discontinuation, we consider the risk of relapse to be too high in most circumstances. Relapse may also be associated with higher overall doses of medication or multiple medications.

Treating with the lowest effective dose of lithium may therefore be an option, as may slowly tapering the dose (over 2 to 4 weeks or longer). If lithium is to be continued, plasma levels need to be monitored closely throughout pregnancy because dose increases are invariably required. Monthly monitoring of lithium plasma levels, U & Es and TFTs should occur in the first half of the pregnancy with more frequent monitoring after that. In late pregnancy lithium levels should perhaps be monitored weekly. To lower peak plasma levels it may also be better to split the total daily dose into three or more doses a day. Dose increases are often required because, in pregnancy, the woman will have an increased volume of distribution and increased renal clearance. As volume changes at delivery and dehydration can occur it has been suggested by some that the lithium dose should be reduced by about 25% to 30% on the estimated day before delivery. As women often do not give birth on their estimated day of delivery, others have suggested hydration or dose reduction of 50% or to pre-pregnancy doses on the day of delivery. Maternal serum monitoring and adequate hydration needs to occur after delivery.

Neonatal adverse effects that have been reported include a 'floppy infant' syndrome characterised by cyanosis and hypertonicity, non-toxic goitre, hypothyroidism, nephrogenic diabetes insipidus and cardiac arrhythmias. *For more information on lithium in pregnancy see Llewellyn et al. 1998 and Yonkers et al. 1998.*

✳ Most data concerning *carbamazepine* and *sodium valproate* use in pregnancy have involved their use in women being treated for epilepsy. They are considered teratogenic and both are associated with neural tube defects with reports of the risk for carbamazepine being 0.5% to 1% and for sodium valproate, 1% to 5%. This risk may increase with the use of more than one AED and may be dose related. Dividing the total daily dose so as to lower peak plasma levels is therefore recommended.

Folic acid has been shown to help prevent neural tube defects and a dose of 4mg/day is recommended in the UK when there has been a previous child born with neural tube defects or if there is a family history. Therefore, even though there are no studies looking at the use of folic acid in women taking carbamazepine and sodium valproate, it has been suggested that folic acid be taken at a dose of 4mg/day (only 5mg is available in the UK) by women taking these drugs. Folic acid needs to be taken at least one month and perhaps for three months, before conception. RBC folate is a better indication of a patient's folate levels than is serum folate. Folic acid must then be continued for a further three months after conception. Women who are considering becoming pregnant or, as most pregnancies are unplanned, perhaps all women of child-bearing age who are taking carbamazepine or sodium valproate should therefore be taking 4mg of folic acid daily. Women who are not taking carbamazepine or sodium valproate and who are of child-bearing age need only take 400mcg of folic acid daily. In women who become pregnant on sodium valproate or carbamazepine, a high resolution ultrasound scan should be carried out at 18 weeks gestation. Maternal serum alpha-fetoprotein (AFP) levels should also be taken.

Minor anomalies have also been reported, including craniofacial abnormalities – a broad, flat nasal bridge, elongated upper lip, rotated ears and fingernail hypoplasia. With increasing age, these features appear to be less prominent. In one study, IQ was not found to be adversely affected in infants exposed to carbamazepine in utero at 5-year follow-up.

To prevent neonatal haemorrhage, vitamin K (10mg/day) should be administered in the last month of gestation to mothers taking enzyme inducing agents (e.g. carbamazepine, phenytoin, phenobarbitone). Neonates at birth should be given 1mg of Vitamin K.

✳ *Gabapentin* and *lamotrigine* are being increasingly used as mood stabilisers. There are however even fewer data relating to their use in pregnancy. Lamotrigine has not been found to be teratogenic in animal studies.

✳ There are conflicting data concerning an association between *benzodiazepines* and congenital malformations although there have been suggestions of a benzodiazepine embryopathy and an association with an increased risk of facial clefts. As with all drugs, the use of benzodiazepines should be avoided, particularly in the 1st trimester. If this has not been possible it may be prudent to perform a level 2 ultrasonography to rule out visible forms of facial cleft, although only severe forms may be visualised. Prolonged use of the drugs has resulted in symptoms of neonatal withdrawal and the use of high doses close to delivery has been associated with a characteristic 'floppy infant syndrome' which includes symptoms such as hypotonia, respiratory embarrassment, hypothermia and difficulty in suckling. If a benzodiazepine is considered to be essential it should be given on a short-term basis at the minimum effective dose. There is most information for *diazepam*, *lorazepam* and *chlordiazepoxide*.

✳   *ECT* is not thought to be teratogenic in pregnancy, based on a limited number of case reports; foetal monitoring is required.

✳   If a simple hypnotic is required, *promethazine* may be safe and appropriate.

Psychotropic Group	Recommended Drugs*
Antidepressants	Nortriptyline Amitriptyline Imipramine Fluoxetine
Antipsychotics	Trifluoperazine Chlorpromazine ? Haloperidol
Sedatives	Promethazine
Mood stabilisers	Lithium, carbamazepine and sodium valproate are best avoided during the first trimester. Folic acid 4mg (5mg) should be given to all women of child-bearing age on carbamazepine and sodium valproate.

●   *There are too few data to make firm recommendations for safe drug use in pregnancy. However, the cited recommendations represent the drugs for which there is the most information available.*

Lactation

General rules

❖ All psychotropic drugs pass into breast-milk. Generally drug concentrations in breast milk are approximately 1% of the maternal plasma level.

❖ There have been few systematic studies performed in breast-feeding mothers. Most of the literature relies on single case presentations.

❖ It is not known what long-term effects there are on the developing infant's CNS.

❖ All drugs should be avoided if the infant was born premature or has renal, hepatic, cardiac or neurological impairment. The infant's hepatic and renal function should be checked before being breast-fed by the mother who is prescribed psychotropic medication.

❖ In general older drugs are preferred as there are more data on their safe use.

❖ It is best to avoid sedating drugs and drugs with long half-lives.

❖ Monoamine oxidase inhibitors (MAOIs) and lithium should be avoided. Also best to avoid clozapine because of the risk of neutropenia.

❖ Generally and if possible, the drug should be given as a single daily dose before the infant's longest sleep period. Breast-feeding should occur immediately before the dose is due. If possible, avoid breast-feeding when drug concentrations peak in milk where this is known (eg. amitriptyline, 1.5 hours; imipramine, 1 hour; moclobemide, < 3 hours; sertraline, 7-10 hours; and chlorpromazine, 2 hours after oral administration).

❖ If the mother was taking the drug during pregnancy, the amount of drug that the infant will be exposed to via breast-feeding will be considerably less than what they were exposed to in utero.

❖ The mother should be continued on the same drug postpartum as was taken during pregnancy.

❖ Monitor the infant for adverse effects: e.g. sedation, irritability

❖ Monitor the infant's development and have a paediatrician check the infant.

❖ Treat the mother with the lowest effective dose as adverse-effects in the infant are often dose-related.

❖ As a general rule, the mother should not breast-feed if she requires a dose of haloperidol > 20mg/day or chlorpromazine > 200mg/day.

❖ Adverse effects in infants have been noted when more than one psychotropic is prescribed. Breast-feeding is therefore best avoided in these situations.

❖ *For more information see Yoshida et al. (1999).*

Psychotropic Group	Recommended drugs
Antidepressants	If medication was taken during pregnancy, continue with this same medication postpartum. If medication is being prescribed for the first time postpartum: Prefer TCAs (except doxepin); Less experience with SSRIs ***Avoid MAOIs***
Antipsychotics	If medication was taken during pregnancy, continue with this same medication postpartum. If medication is being prescribed for the first time postpartum: Few data available. Most data for chlorpromazine, haloperidol and trifluoperazine but monitor the infant closely for adverse effects and avoid polytherapy. Few data on atypical antipsychotics
Mood Stabilisers	Carbamazepine Sodium Valproate ***Avoid lithium***

Medical Co-morbidity

Cardiovascular Disease

General principles:

❖   Thorough physical history and examination are fundamental to all good medical and pharmacological management.

❖   Polypharmacy with psychotropic drugs should ideally be avoided at all times, but particularly in the presence of cardiac disease.

❖   Beware of interactions with drugs producing changes in cardiac rate and in electrolyte balance.

❖   The elderly are at higher risk of virtually all common cardiac pathologies.

❖   Some drugs are specifically contraindicated and should be avoided e.g. pimozide. Sertindole has recently been withdrawn, except for use on a named-patient basis because of its cardiac effects and reports of sudden death – its use in cardiac patients should be considered an absolute contraindication.

❖   Avoid rapid escalation of drug doses in established cardiac disease.

Where cardiovascular disease is established, the need for starting a psychotropic drug should be reviewed in light of cardiac medications already prescribed. However, the incidence of some psychiatric illness is increased in the context of cardiac disease. For example, myocardial infarction (MI) is associated with an increased incidence of depressive illness; this in turn adversely affects the mortality post MI and should therefore be actively treated.

Specific clinical situations:

Myocardial infarction

❖   Avoid all antidepressants if possible for two months after MI. If required (see above) use SSRIs (except fluvoxamine and citalopram, which may be more cardiotoxic in overdose) or mianserin. Avoid tricyclics. If a sedative antidepressant is required, use trazodone or nefazodone (beware hypotension).

❖   Avoid high dose antipsychotics. In addition to orthostatic hypotension and tachycardia, most antipsychotics have direct cardiac muscle depressant effects. This toxicity is most common with high dosing and in damaged cardiac muscle post MI. Generally, phenothiazines are more hypotensive than butyrophenones. Avoid pimozide in a patient with any cardiac abnormality in the history. Clozapine should be started slowly and with caution less than a year post MI or in cardiac disease. Olanzapine may be a safe alternative in the acute post MI, as it only rarely causes hypotension.

Heart failure

❖   This may be acute or chronic. If chronic and stable, avoid drugs known to alter cardiac function, e.g. beta- blockers. Be cautious with those producing orthostatic hypotension e.g. clozapine and risperidone or tricyclics, nefazodone and trazodone. Drugs producing fluid retention, such as carbamazepine, should also be avoided or used with caution.

❖   If acute, the cause of the heart failure will determine which drugs are safe to use. Some hypotensive effects of psychotropics may be beneficial, especially in the context of hypertensive, high output failure. If the myocardium is unstable, it may be necessary for cardiotoxic psychotropic medication to be discontinued or avoided until the heart is stabilised.

❖   Use great caution with lithium and changes in diuretic therapy.

Angina

❖   Avoid drugs causing orthostatic hypotension. This may exacerbate angina by producing rebound tachycardia.

❖   Phenothiazines, clozapine and risperidone amongst others can all cause tachycardia and should be used with caution.

❖   Most antidepressants are thought to be safe in angina, but trazodone, nefazodone and tricyclics should usually be avoided.

Hypertension

❖   Psychotropic drugs may interact with prescribed antihypertensive medication in a beneficial or dangerous manner. Orthostatic effects of psychotropic medication should be monitored closely. Patients should be monitored initially if choosing drugs with known hypotensive effects. Choice of treatment should take into account the duration of the hypertension and the state of the myocardium.

❖ Sometimes the lower doses of tricyclics and antipsychotics can produce rebound hypertensive pressor responses on initiation of treatment. Avoid pimozide. Note also some dangerous interactions between some antidepressants and archaic antihypertensives (adrenergic neurone blockers).

❖ Note the possible occurrence of hypertension with clozapine and high dose venlafaxine.

Arrhythmias

For depression, SSRIs are the drugs of first choice. Note that fluvoxamine and citalopram have weak associations with cardiac arrhythmias.

In psychosis, use sulpiride or olanzapine, but avoid phenothiazines, butyrophenones and especially pimozide. Sertindole is an absolute contraindication in cardiac arrhythmias.

For treatment of comorbid anxiety, it is important to differentiate between cardiac arrhythmias and panic disorder; 24 hour halter monitoring may be useful if the diagnosis is in doubt.

Notes on Some Specific Drugs:

Lithium is contraindicated in cardiac failure and in sick sinus syndrome. Lithium commonly causes flattening of T-waves and T-wave inversion. Widening of the QRS complex has also been reported. In healthy patients a baseline ECG with yearly follow-up is desirable, although the T-wave changes are felt to be benign and often disappear with continued therapy. In patients with cardiac disease closer monitoring may be indicated. It should be used with caution in patients with pre-existing conduction abnormalities. The usual precautions and care should be exercised when prescribing with other drugs. Note the important interaction with diuretics.

Benzodiazepines are generally safe, but should be avoided in pulmonary insufficiency and acute or chronic pulmonary failure, which may be more common in heart disease. Avoid chlormethiazole in pulmonary insufficiency.

Disulfuram is contraindicated in cardiac failure, hypertensive heart disease and can produce cardiac arrest in an antabuse reaction. Best avoided.

Lofexidine should be used with caution post MI and in cardiac disease.

91
Hepatic Impairment

General Rules

◆ The severity of liver disease, rather than its aetiology, relates more directly to the impairment of drug metabolism. The risk of drug toxicity thus increases with the severity of the disease and in fulminant hepatic failure, drugs must be used with great care. In cholestasis, however, drug toxicity tends to be less of a problem.

◆ Clinical signs of hepatic impairment include: jaundice, ascites, encephalopathy, hypoalbuminaemia and a prolonged prothrombin time.

◆ Liver function tests are not strictly quantitative and do not correlate well with impairment of drug metabolism. It is therefore impossible to predict to what extent a drug's metabolism will be affected. In general, however, the more abnormal the liver function tests, the more severe the liver impairment and the lower the starting dose of psychotropic that should be used.

◆ Portal-systemic shunting, which may be associated with oesophageal varices, fetor hepaticus or hepatic encephalopathy, allows increased systemic availability of drugs. This is important for drugs with a high (>50%) first-pass clearance by the liver and thus they should be prescribed at lower doses.

◆ Patients with liver disease may be more sensitive to type A (predictable) adverse effects of drugs even at 'therapeutic levels'.

◆ In severe liver disease, sedative drugs and drugs which cause constipation may adversely affect cerebral function and may precipitate or unmask hepatic encephalopathy. Over half of patients with cirrhosis demonstrate subclinical encephalopathy on neuropsychological or neurophysiological testing, despite having no overt neuropsychiatric symptoms.

◆ In even moderate liver disease renal function may be affected. Lower doses of renally cleared drugs may therefore be required.

◆ All psychotropics should be started at a low dose and dose adjustments should be made slowly. The total dose of psychotropic should generally be lower than that considered normal.

Psychotropics

◆ There are few clinical studies on the use of psychotropics in liver disease.

◆ Most psychotropics are extensively metabolised by the liver. Therefore in liver disease psychotropic plasma levels will be increased. *Amisulpride, sulpiride, lithium* and *gabapentin* undergo no or minimal hepatic metabolism.

◆ Drugs which are highly protein bound - *TCAs, SSRIs* (except *citalopram), nefazodone, reboxetine, trazodone* and antipsychotics (except *amisulpride* and *sulpiride*) - may have increased free plasma levels. Changes such as these will not show up in measured (total) plasma levels.

♦ Drugs with a high first-pass clearance by the liver – eg. *imipramine, amitriptyline, desipramine, doxepin, haloperidol* – should be started at lower doses than usual.

♦ *Phenothiazines* (especially *chlorpromazine)* and the irreversible *MAOIs* are hepatotoxic and should be avoided.

♦ If a psychotropic is added, liver function tests must be monitored weekly. If any individual parameter rises 2-3 times above baseline, withdrawal of the drug would be necessary.

Antidepressants

■ With respect to the antidepressants, there is perhaps most safe clinical use with imipramine. *Lofepramine* is contraindicated and the more sedative TCAs such as *amitriptyline* and *dothiepin* are best avoided.

■ There is less clinical experience with the newer antidepressants in liver disease, although it has been suggested that in depressed patients with a history of alcohol abuse the non-sedating SSRIs would appear preferable to TCAs. There have been published studies with *fluoxetine, paroxetine, sertraline, moclobemide* and *nefazodone* in patients with cirrhosis. The drugs' half-lives were increased and clearance reduced and so lower doses should be employed in clinically significant liver disease.

■ In well-compensated cirrhotic patients, the dose of *fluoxetine* should be reduced by at least 50%. In more severe liver disease, a greater reduction would be needed.

■ In a single dose study, pharmacokinetic data for *paroxetine* in patients with liver disease was similar to healthy volunteers and for this reason it has been suggested to be the SSRI of first choice. Higher plasma concentrations and reduced elimination have been seen in a 14 day multiple dose study and so it is recommended that doses at the lower end of the dose range should be used.

■ The elimination half-life of *sertraline* is significantly prolonged and, as it is contraindicated in liver disease in the data sheet, it should be avoided.

■ For *moclobemide*, the dose should be reduced by one-half to two-thirds.

■ Patients with liver disease may be exposed to higher concentrations of *nefazodone* and its metabolites and so a lower daily dose should be used.

■ Minimal data exist for *citalopram* although the manufacturer recommends that doses should be restricted to the lower end of the dose range in liver disease.

■ *Mirtazapine's* clearance is reduced in moderate to severe hepatic impairment and the dose should therefore be titrated cautiously.

■ *Reboxetine* undergoes extensive hepatic metabolism and thus the dose should be started at 2mg twice daily and increased according to efficacy and tolerability.

■ Data on file for *venlafaxine* suggest that in mild liver disease (PT 14 secs) no dose reduction is required while in moderate liver impairment (PT 14-18 secs), venlafaxine's dose should be reduced by 50% which can be given once a day. There are too few data to support its use in severe liver disease.

Antipsychotics

❖ *Haloperidol* is often considered the antipsychotic of choice in liver disease or if there has been a history of drug-induced hepatotoxicity.

❖ *Sulpiride* may also be an appropriate choice. Only 5% of the drug is metabolised by the liver, although there have been occasional reports of liver toxicity.

❖ Few problems have been reported with *flupenthixol* and *zuclopenthixol* and so they may also be options.

❖ As *amisulpride* is predominately renally excreted, a dose reduction is not necessary. On theoretical grounds it may therefore be an appropriate choice in hepatic impairment but we await more data before it can be recommended.

❖ Lower doses of *clozapine* are required and plasma levels should be obtained, as there is some evidence that these relate to efficacy and adverse effects. A plasma level of 350mg/l should be aimed for. (Note that clozapine has been linked to toxic hepatitis).

❖ Doses of up to 7.5mg of *olanzapine* have been administered safely to subjects with hepatic dysfunction. However, increased hepatic transaminase levels have been reported, which may complicate monitoring.

❖ *Quetiapine* is extensively metabolised with plasma clearance being reduced in subjects with hepatic impairment (stable alcoholic cirrhosis). The manufacturer recommends a starting dose of 25mg in hepatic impairment, which is increased in increments of 25 – 50mg according to efficacy and tolerability.

❖ *Risperidone* should be started at 0.5mg bd and increased to a maximum of 4mg/day.

❖ *Sertindole* is contraindicated in severe liver disease.

❖ *Zotepine* should be prescribed with caution in patients with hepatic impairment. The dose should be started at 25mg twice daily and increased gradually according to efficacy and tolerability to a maximum of 75mg twice daily. LFTs should be monitored weekly for the at least the first three months.

Mood Stabilisers

❑ *Valproate* has been associated with liver toxicity and so is contraindicated in severe liver disease and must be used with caution in mild-moderate impairment.

❏   *Carbamazepine* must also be used with caution in hepatic disease.

❏   *Lamotrigine* is contraindicated when there is significant hepatic impairment.

❏   *Lithium* and perhaps *gabapentin* are thus the mood stabilisers of choice in liver disease.

Anxiolytics

❖   If an anxiolytic is required, a short acting *benzodiazepine* at a low dose is recommended. If *chlormethiazole* is required, it should be commenced at one-third the standard dose. Chlormethiazole may be useful in the severely agitated patient who may be aggressive. It must be remembered that sedative drugs can precipitate hepatic encephalopathy or coma in patients with liver disease and so these drugs should be used cautiously.

Psychotropic classification	Recommended drugs
Antidepressants	Imipramine [10mg tds (od in the elderly) for 2 weeks, then increase by 10mg each week until a therapeutic effect is seen] Paroxetine (low dose)
Antipsychotics	Haloperidol (low dose) Sulpiride
Mood stabilisers	Lithium ?Gabapentin*
Anxiolytics	Lorazepam Oxazepam (Use low dose)

*Limited data for use as a mood stabiliser. It is not licensed for this use.

Renal Impairment

General Rules

Assessment of renal function is normally made by calculating the creatinine clearance (CrCl). The CrCl is predicted using a single measurement of serum creatinine and formulae such as that of Cockroft and Gault. The formula gives a good estimate of the glomerular filtration rate (GFR).

$$CrCl = \frac{y\ (140 - age)\ x\ IBW}{serum\ creatinine}$$

CrCl = ml/min

y = 1.04 (females) or 1.23 (males)

IBW = kg
= 50 kg + 2.3 kg per inch over 5 foot (males)
= 45.5 kg + 2.3 kg per inch over 5 foot (females)

serum creatinine = mmol/l

This equation assumes that renal function is stable. The accuracy of the test is poor in patients with a GFR < 20ml/min, in debilitated patients and in overweight patients (use IBW).

Renal impairment is divided into three grades:

Grade	GFR	Serum Creatinine
Mild	20-50 ml/min	120-200 mmol/l
Moderate	10-20 ml/min	200-400 mmol/l
Severe	< 10ml/min	> 400 mmol/l

❖ The extent of accumulation of drugs given to patients with renal impairment depends on the degree of renal dysfunction and the dose. Consequently, before an appropriate drug or dose schedule can be chosen the severity of renal impairment must be assessed.

❖ Renal function declines with age. Because many of the elderly will have reduced body mass, their GFR will be less than 50 ml/min even though their serum creatinine may not be raised. It may therefore be best to assume at least mild renal impairment in the elderly.

❖ Renal impairment is an important consideration when drugs are primarily cleared by the kidney or when metabolites are pharmacologically active or toxic and are dependent on the kidney for elimination.

❖ All antidepressants and antipsychotics (with the exception of amisulpride and sulpiride) are predominatly metabolised by the liver. Generally only small amounts are excreted unchanged in the urine. The drugs may have active metabolites that are excreted renally.

❖ All psychotropics should be started at a low dose and dose adjustments should be made according to tolerability and efficacy. The drug may need to be given in divided doses. Plasma levels may be useful.

❖　　　　Adverse effects such as postural hypotension and confusion may be more frequent in patients with renal disease. This may be because of fluid volume deficits, dialysis, autonomic insufficiency, concomitant anti-hypertensive medication or metabolic cerebral impairment. Excessive sedation can also occur frequently in patients with renal failure.

❖　　　　Psychotropics with anticholinergic activity may cause urinary retention and interfere with precise urine measurements. The aliphatic and piperidine phenothiazines, *chlorpromazine* and *thioridazine*, and the tricyclic antidepressants, *amitriptyline* and *imipramine*, are more likely to cause these problems.

❖　　　　There is little information about the dialysability of antipsychotics. Because they are lipid soluble, have large volumes of distribution and are highly protein bound, most would not expect to be cleared by dialysis. This is also true for the antidepressants.

Antidepressants

◆　　　　The metabolites of *tricyclic antidepressants* are excreted by the kidneys and accumulation may occur causing an increase in adverse effects eg. hypotension, sedation, and anticholinergic effects. Tricyclics should be started at a low dose and increased slowly according to tolerability and efficacy and the dose should be divided. Up to 50% of the dose of lofepramine is excreted unchanged by the kidneys and is best avoided in severe renal failure, although low doses have been used by patients on dialysis.

◆　　　　Approximately 13% of *citalopram* is excreted unchanged in the urine and 20% is excreted as metabolites, some of which are pharmacologically active. There are no data on the use of citalopram in moderate to severe renal failure (ie. CrCl < 20ml/min). Dose adjustment is not considered necessary in mild renal failure.

◆　　　　In a multiple dose study, 20 mg of *fluoxetine* was given daily for more than 60 days to depressed patients with normal renal function and to renally-impaired, depressed patients who required haemodialysis. Steady state concentrations of fluoxetine in the dialysis patients were almost twice that of those with normal renal function. In mild to moderate renal failure, fluoxetine should be commenced at 10 mg a day or 20 mg every second day and increased only if necessary. The use of fluoxetine in severe renal failure is contraindicated by the manufacturer but in practice it is often used.

◆　　　　Pharmacokinetic data for the use of *fluvoxamine* in renal impairment are not available. The manufacturers recommend that treatment should be begun with a low dose and the patient carefully monitored.

◆　　　　In a single dose study, the mean maximum plasma concentration and half-life of *paroxetine* increased as renal function decreased. There was however wide inter-subject variability and paroxetine was well tolerated by all subjects. There have been no multiple-dose studies and there are no data on the use of paroxetine in depressed patients with a creatinine clearance less than

5ml/minute or in renal dialysis. It is highly protein bound and therefore unlikely to be removed by dialysis and additional dosing after dialysis is not necessary. Because of limited data we recommend that paroxetine be started at 10mg/day and increased only if necessary according to tolerability and efficacy. The maximum dose should be towards the lower end of the range recommended for the general population. (Liquid preparation now available.)

◆ In a single-dose study, 100mg of *sertraline* was administered to patients with a CrCl < 20ml/min and a control group. There were no differences in pharmacokinetic values but steady state pharmacokinetic data are not available. As sertraline has an active metabolite and as there are limited data, it should be used with caution in renal failure.

◆ There are limited data on the use of *MAOIs* in renal impairment but one reference suggests that dose reductions are not required for phenelzine.

◆ Less then 1% of *moclobemide* and approximately 6-10% of the N-oxide metabolite, which may be active, is cleared renally. In patients with different grades of renal impairment, single-dose studies showed that pharmacokinetic data do not vary amongst the group. The manufacturer recommends that dose reductions are not necessary in renal failure.

◆ *Mirtazapine's* clearance is reduced in moderate to severe renal impairment and so dose adjustments may be required.

◆ Limited data exist on the use of *nefazodone* in renal impairment. Nefazodone is metabolised hepatically to active metabolites and with chronic administration accumulation may occur in patients with severe renal impairment. Lower doses should be used.

◆ *Reboxetine's* half-life is increased approximately two-fold in patients with renal impairment. The manufacturer recommends a starting dose of 2mg twice daily which can be increased depending on patient response.

◆ In renal failure, *venlafaxine* clearance is reduced by up to 55%. If CrCl > 30ml/min no dose adjustment is required. If CrCl is 10-30 ml/min, the daily dose should be reduced by 50% and may be given once a day if tolerated. Few data exist for patients with severe renal impairment and its use is not recommended. In haemodialysis patients, however, venlafaxine has been given at half the normal dose.

Antipsychotics

✶ *Chlorpromazine* has many active metabolites and renal excretion is slow. There have been reports of chlorpromazine metabolite accumulation leading to toxic psychosis and hallucinations. Because it causes sedation, postural hypotension and anticholinergic adverse effects, its use should be avoided.

✶ There are few data on the use of *thioridazine* in renal failure. However as thioridazine has been associated with irreversible pigmentary retinopathy at doses greater than 600mg/day, as it causes postural hypotension and anticholinergic adverse effects and because it has active metabolites it is best to avoid its use in renal failure.

✱ *Trifluoperazine*, a piperazine antipsychotic, is less likely to cause sedation, postural hypotension and anticholinergic adverse effects than aliphatic and piperidine phenothiazines. Few data exist on its use in renal failure but a starting dose of 4mg/day has been suggested.

✱ In severe renal impairment there may be some accumulation of the metabolites of *flupenthixol* and *zuclopenthixol*. As these have little pharmacological effect a dose reduction should not be necessary.

✱ Few data exist on the use of *haloperidol* in renal failure. In a 48 year old patient with chronic renal failure up to 4 mg of haloperidol was safely given intravenously over a thirty minute period. In an elderly patient with end-stage renal disease haloperidol was given in doses of 2-4mg/day. In a second elderly patient with moderate chronic renal failure, it was suggested that higher plasma concentrations than expected were obtained from a dose of 4 mg/day. Accumulation may therefore occur. Thus, even though some have suggested no dose adjustments in renal failure others have proposed that haloperidol be initiated at low doses e.g. 1mg/day. Haloperidol is less sedative and anticholinergic and less likely to cause postural hypotension than chlorpromazine.

✱ *Amisulpride* is eliminated by the renal route. When GFR is between 30-60 ml/min, the dose should be halved and when GFR is between 10 – 30 ml/min, the dose should be reduced to a third. There are no data when GFR is <10 ml/min and so care is needed and amisulpride should probably be avoided.

✱ *Clozapine* causes marked postural hypotension, sedation and anticholinergic effects. It is contraindicated in severe renal disease. In mild to moderate renal failure, the dose should be commenced at 12.5mg and then increased slowly in small increments.

✱ *Olanzapine* 5 mg was administered to subjects with moderate or severe renal failure and to healthy subjects in an open-label, fixed-dose study. Adverse effects seen were similar between the groups, although asthenia appeared more frequently in the renally impaired subjects. Their renal status may however have predisposed them to the asthenia. Overall females experienced more adverse effects. The pharmacokinetics of olanzapine in subjects with severe renal failure compared with those subjects with normal renal function was similar. The protein binding of olanzapine was not affected by renal disease. It has therefore been suggested that the dose of olanzapine will not change in renal failure. However, as there are few data on its use in renal failure, olanzapine should be commenced at 5 mg a day and increased according to tolerability and efficacy.

✱ *Quetiapine* has not been studied in clinically relevant doses in patients with renal impairment. The manufacturer recommends starting at 25mg/day and increasing in increments of 25 – 50mg to an effective dose.

✱ Approximately 40% of the dose of 9-hydroxy-risperidone, the active metabolite of *risperidone*, is renally excreted. In renal failure, clearance of 9-hydroxy-risperidone is reduced while its elimination half-life is increased. Clearance of the active fraction, which consists of risperidone and 9-hydroxy-risperidone, is also reduced by about 50% in patients with renal disease. Experience with this drug in renal failure is limited but a starting dose of 0.5 mg twice a day, increasing up to a maximum dose of 2 mg twice a day is recommended.

✶   *Sertindole* may cause significant postural hypotension, but has the advantage in this population of being less sedating and less anticholinergic. Its clearance is not greatly affected by renal impairment, but experience is limited in renal failure. Sertindole is contraindicated with drugs that prolong the QT interval or predispose to hypokalaemia and ECG monitoring is necessary. Only named-patient use is allowed.

✶   As *sulpiride* is primarily excreted by the kidneys, the dose may need to be decreased or the dosage interval increased according to the level of renal impairment. The following changes have been recommended.

CrCl (ml/min)	Dose adjustment	Dose interval
30-60	70%	x 1.5
10-30	50%	x 2
<10	34%	x3

There is no information on whether sulpiride or its conjugates are dialysable but binding to plasma protein is low (14-40%).

✶   In renal impairment, *zotepine* should be started at 25mg twice daily, with the dose increased gradually to a maximum of 75mg twice daily.

Mood Stabilisers/Antiepileptic Drugs

❋   *Lithium* is contraindicated by the manufacturer in renal insufficiency. If it is considered necessary, 50-75% of the usual dose has been recommended in mild to moderate renal failure and 25-50% of the usual dose in severe renal failure. Lithium plasma levels would need to be checked frequently. Therapeutic plasma levels have been obtained when lithium has been given at a dose of 600mg three times a week after haemodialysis.

❋   Approximately 1-2% of unchanged *carbamazepine* and its 10-11 epoxide metabolite are excreted in the urine. There are no pharmacokinetic data in patients with renal impairment but, because there is minimal renal excretion, dose adjustments have not generally been considered necessary, although some suggest a reduction of 25% in severe renal impairment. Serum levels should, at any rate, be monitored.

❋   Less than 4% of *valproic acid* is excreted unchanged in the urine. It has numerous metabolites, some of which are active. It has been suggested that dose adjustments are not necessary in renal impairment but free serum valproic acid levels should be monitored as protein binding is affected and free levels may increase dramatically at times.

❋   If *gabapentin* is used in renal impairment, its dose must be reduced according to the following:

Creatinine Clearance	Dose
60-90 ml/min	400 mg tds
30-60 ml/min	300 mg bd
15-30 ml/min	300 mg daily
<15 ml/min	300 mg alternate days

✳   Single-dose studies of *lamotrigine* have not shown any change in serum concentrations. Lamotrigine should, however, still be used with caution in renal failure as there may be accumulation of its glucuronide metabolite.

✳   *Carbamazepine* and *valproate* are preferred to *lithium* as mood stabilisers. They are also preferred over *lamotrigine* and *gabapentin* , having much more data relating to efficacy and safety as mood stabilisers.

✳   *Benzodiazepines* may accumulate in renal failure and this should be accounted for in dosing.

Psychotropic Classification	Recommended Drugs
Antidepressants	Tricyclic antidepressants eg. amitriptyline – initially 25mg/day and increase by 25mg/week according to tolerability and response. The daily dose should be divided initially. SSRIs Most clinical experience with fluoxetine/paroxetine – start at 10mg/day
Antipsychotics	Start at low dose and increase according to tolerability and efficacy. Haloperidol eg. 1mg/day Trifluoperazine eg. 4mg/day Flupenthixol eg. 3mg/day Zuclopenthixol eg. 10mg/day
Mood stabilisers	Carbamazepine 100mg BD and increase after 1 week to 200mg BD. (Aim for a Cp > 7mg/1) Sodium Valproate 500mg MR/day (Aim for a Cp > 50mg/1)

Psychiatric Effects of Medical Therapies

❖ Drug-induced psychiatric dysfunction is an important consideration in the differential diagnosis of medical patients with psychiatric co-morbidity. Such effects are common and may relate to direct or indirect CNS toxicity due to the specific agent, pharmacokinetic or pharmacodynamic interactions with psychotropics or with other medical therapies or to interactions with the patient's underlying medical or psychiatric diagnosis.

❖ Psychiatric illness often goes undiagnosed in patients with medical co-morbidity, particularly in a hospital setting. The effects of illness or of drugs may alter the presentation.

❖ The clinician must be aware of both the effects of medical therapies on psychiatric presentation as well as the effects of psychotropics on the patient's medical condition and the potential for drug interactions between the two. For example, MAOIs and moclobemide are contraindicated in phaeochromocytoma and hyperthyroidism (tranylcypramine and moclobemide) and lithium may be contraindicated in hypothyroidism and Addison's disease. In GI illness, SSRIs may exacerbate nausea while tricyclics and other anticholinergics may exacerbate constipation and their levels may be increased by concomitant use of cimetidine. In prostatic hypertrophy, tricyclics and other agents with anticholinergic properties can cause urinary retention and, in narrow angle glaucoma, they are contraindicated as they may precipitate an acute crisis. MAOIs are not recommended in the elderly, congestive heart failure, and after CVAs. Tricyclics are contraindicated in heart block and following myocardial infarction. Prescribing of psychotropics in renal disease, liver impairment, cardiac illness and in neuropsychiatric conditions is discussed in other sections of these guidelines.

❖ Drug interactions frequently exacerbate both the psychiatric symptoms and the medical condition. CNS toxicity may develop from lithium and sumatriptan in a person with migraine, for example, or from fluoxetine and selegiline in Parkinson's disease presenting with a confusion state. The common analgesic dextropropoxyphene frequently causes serious interactions with many drugs such as carbamazepine, increasing levels precipitously. Such interactions affecting care need not be pharmacokinetic only. Psychotropics causing postural hypotension may have additive effects with diuretics. In patients with agranulocytosis or with marrow suppression from chemotherapeutic agents, tricyclics, mianserin, carbamazepine and clozapine are all contraindicated. Drug interactions with warfarin, antiepileptic drugs, cardiac medications and psychotropics are further discussed in other sections of these guidelines.

❖ Many agents have been implicated in causing *delirium and cognitive impairment*. Of the cardiovascular medications, beta-blockers have been most implicated in producing depression, an acute confusional state, hallucinosis, sleep disruption and chronic fatigue symptoms. These risks are not, however as great as originally feared. Digoxin, quinidine, disopyramide, clonidine, methyldopa and others may also cause acute confusional states and/or cognitive impairment. Anticholinergics, tricyclic antidepressants, and antihistamines frequently cause delirium, particularly in the elderly. Antiparkinson agents and nonsteroidal anti-inflammatory drugs (NSAIDs) have also been implicated.

❖ *Anxiety* may be caused by stimulant use or abuse and is most common with caffeinism. Ten to 15% of patients receiving dopaminergic agents will experience anxiety as an adverse effect. Thyroxine, various cardiac drugs, theophylline and sympathomimetics may also cause anxiety. The elderly may have a paradoxical excitement with associated anxiety with benzodiazepines, barbiturates and other sedative-hypnotics. The withdrawal effects of sedative-hypnotics frequently precipitate anxiety.

❖ *Depression* may be caused by many agents, including propranolol, digoxin (particularly in the elderly), methyldopa, corticosteroids, NSAIDs, cimetidine, antipsychotics and others.

❖ *Mania and/or psychosis* have been reported with digoxin, quinidine, procainamide, disopyramide, corticosteroids, NSAIDs, antiparkinsonian agents, cimetidine and many other medical therapies. Some of the major psychiatric effects of medical therapies are listed in the following table (Modified from McConnell and Duffy, 1994).

Drug	Psychiatric Effects
Antihypertensive Drugs	
Clonidine	depression, mania, agitation
Propranolol	depression, mania, delirium, psychosis
Nifedipine	depression
Captopril	mania, agitation
Antiarrhythmics	
Procainamide	depression, mania, delirium, psychosis
Lignocaine	depression, delirium, psychosis
Disopyramide	delirium, psychosis
Antimicrobial Agents	
Penicillins	depression, agitation, visual hallucinations
Tetracycline	depression, hallucinations
Cephalosporins	delirium, psychosis
Antimalarials	psychosis, visual hallucinations
Antiparkinson Drugs	
Anticholinergics	delirium, psychosis, visual hallucinations, dementia
Amantadine	depression, agitation, delirium, psychosis, visual hallucinations
Levodopa	depression, mania, anxiety, agitation, psychosis, visual hallucinations, delirium, cognitive impairment

Antihistamines	
H1 blockers (diphenhydramine)	delirium
H2 blockers (cimetidine)	depression, mania, delirium, psychosis, visual hallucinations
Antineoplastic Drugs	
Interferon	depression, agitation, delirium
Vincristine	depression
C- asparaginase	depression, delirium, psychosis
Endocrine Agents	
Corticosteroids	depression, mania, psychosis, delirium
Oral contraceptives	depression
Thyroxine	anxiety, agitation, mania, psychosis, visual hallucinations
Antiepileptic Drugs	
Barbiturates (phenobarbitone primidone)	hyperactivity (esp. in children), sedation, sexual dysfunction, aggression, learning deficits, cognitive impairment, depression, personality change; Positive effects: anxiolytic/hypnotic
Benzodiazepines (clonazepam, diazepam)	aggression, confusion, depression, disinhibition, irritability, cognitive impairment; Positive effects: anxiolytic/hypnotic; antimanic (clonazepam)
Carbamazepine	depression, irritability, sexual dysfunction, mania; Positive effects: antidepressant, antimanic, treatment of aggression and bipolar disorder
Clobazam	similar side effect profile to other benzodiazepines but may have lower overall incidence of cognitive and behavioural side effects; ?Anxiolytic/positive psychotropic effects
Gabapentin	sedation, ataxia, aggression and hyperactivity (children); few drug interactions; ? positive psychotropic effects
Hydantoins (phenytoin)	sedation, ataxia, dementia, affective disorder, confusion, cognitive impairment, progressive encephalopathy; Positive effects: ? antiaggressive, ?anxiolytic effects
Lamotrigine	may have additive toxicity when used with carbamazepine, ataxia, dizziness; ? positive psychotropic effects
Succinimides (ethosuximide, methsuximide)	psychosis ("alternating psychosis" – adolescents, young adults), drowsiness, insomnia, irritability, ? cognitive effects, personality change ; Positive effects: improvement in attention / concentration (likely related to seizure improvement)
Tiagabine	? depression, psychosis, ? anxiolytic effects, ? effects in tardive dyskinesia
Topiramate	sedation, confusion, cognitive dysfunction, asthenia
Valproate	progressive encephalopathy, dementia, depression, extrapyramidal effects; Positive effects: antimanic, treatment of aggression and bipolar disorder
Vigabatrin	depression, psychosis

Neuropsychiatric Conditions

I) Alcohol and Substance Misuse

Prescribing for Alcohol Detoxification

◆   Alcohol withdrawal is associated with significant morbidity and mortality when improperly managed.

◆   Chlordiazepoxide (or a similar benzodiazepine) is the drug of choice in treating alcohol withdrawal symptoms.

◆   Parenteral vitamin replacement is an important adjunctive treatment for the prophylaxis and/or treatment of Wernicke-Korsakoff syndrome and other vitamin-related neuropsychiatric conditions.

◆   The majority of patients can be detoxified in the community. However, in-patient detoxification is indicated where there is:

> A history of delirium tremens or withdrawal seizures
>
> A history of failed community detoxification
>
> Poor social support
>
> Cognitive impairment

Chlordiazepoxide

The approach advocated here is to prescribe chlordiazepoxide according to a flexible regimen over the first 24 hours, with dosage titrated against the rated severity of withdrawal symptoms. This is followed by a fixed 5-day reducing regimen, based upon the dosage requirement estimated during the first 24 hours.

Occasionally (e.g. in delirium tremens (DTs)) the flexible regimen may need to be prolonged beyond the first 24 hours. However, rarely (if ever) is it necessary to resort to the use of other drugs, such as antipsychotics (associated with reduced seizure threshold) or intravenous chlormethiazole (associated with risk of overdose).

The intention of the flexible protocol for the first 24 hours is to titrate dosage of chlordiazepoxide against severity of alcohol withdrawal symptoms. It is necessary to avoid either under-treatment (associated with patient discomfort and a higher incidence of complications such as fits or DTs), or over-treatment (associated with excessive sedation and risk of toxicity/interaction with alcohol consumed prior to admission).

For out-patient detoxification, the dosage will have to be estimated based on clinical judgement and/or known dosage requirements in previous detoxification(s) of the same patient. In the in-patient setting it is possible to be more responsive, with constant monitoring of the severity of withdrawal symptoms, linked to the administered dose of chlordiazepoxide.

Prescribing

First 24 hours (day 1)

On admission, the client should be assessed by a doctor and prescribed chlordiazepoxide. (Diazepam is used in some centres and may be used for those with a history of sensitivity to chlordiazepoxide although some metabolites are shared.) Three doses of chlordiazepoxide must be specified:

First Dose (stat)

This is the first dose of chlordiazepoxide, which will be administered by ward staff immediately following admission, as a fixed 'stat' dose. It should be estimated based upon:

◆ Clinical signs and symptoms of withdrawal (see below)

◆ Breath alcohol concentration (BAC) on admission and 1 hour later.

The dose prescribed should usually be in the range 5-50 mg. However, if withdrawal symptoms on admission are mild, or if the breath alcohol is very high, or if the BAC is rising, the initial dose may be 0 mg (i.e. nothing).

Incremental Dose (range)

This is the range within which subsequent doses of chlordiazepoxide should be administered during the first 24 hours (see below). A dose of 5-40 mg will cover almost all circumstances.

Maximum dose in 24 hours

This is the maximum cumulative dose which may be given during the first 24 hours. It may be estimated according to clinical judgement, but **250 mg should really be adequate for most cases**. Doses above 250mg should not be prescribed without prior discussion with a Consultant or Senior Registrar.

The cumulative chlordiazepoxide dose administered during the initial 24-hour assessment is called the BASELINE DOSE, and this is used to calculate the subsequent reducing regime.

Days 2-5

After the initial 24-hour assessment period, patients are detoxified using a standardised reducing regime. Chlordiazepoxide is given in divided doses four times daily with the afternoon and evening doses proportionately higher. This is to provide night sedation (but note that the effect of chlordiazepoxide and its metabolites is long-lived). The dose should be reduced each day by approximately 20% of the Baseline Dose, so that no chlordiazepoxide is given on day six.

Note:

❖   No chlordiazepoxide should be prescribed on a PRN basis after the initial assessment is complete. Patients exhibiting significant further symptoms may have psychiatric (or other) complications and should be seen by the ward or duty doctor.

❖   A longer regimen may be required in the case of patients who have DTs or a history of DTs. This should be discussed with a Senior Registrar or Consultant, and tailored according to clinical need.

Observations and administration

After chlordiazepoxide has been prescribed as above, the first 'stat' dose is given immediately. Subsequent doses during the first 24 hours are administered with a frequency and dosage which depend upon the observations of alcohol withdrawal status rated by the ward staff.

Observations
      Each set of observations consists of:

◆   Applying an alcohol withdrawal scale (e.g. CIWA-Ar) and/or clinical observation.

◆   Taking BP

◆   Taking Pulse

◆   Alcometer (1st and 2nd observations only).

Observations should be recorded:

I.   During the admission procedure, immediately after the patient has arrived on the ward.

II.   Throughout the first 24 hours, at a frequency depending upon:

◆   Severity of withdrawal

◆   Whether or not chlordiazepoxide has been administered.

III.   Twice daily from days 2-6.

If a patient is asleep (and this is not due to intoxication) she/he should not be woken up for observations. However, it should be recorded that she/he was asleep.

Administration of chlordiazepoxide during first 24 hours.

Chlordiazepoxide should be administered when withdrawal symptoms are considered significant (usually a CIWA-Ar score of more than 15). If a patient suffers hallucinations or agitation, an increased dose of chlordiazepoxide should be administered, according to clinical judgement.

If a patient shows a high Alcometer reading, initial dosage of chlordiazepoxide should be more cautious. However, it is the relative fall in blood alcohol concentration that determines the need for medication, not the absolute figure. (Hence the need to take two Alcometer readings at an interval, soon after admission.)

Relationship between CIWA-Ar score, frequency of continuing observations, and administration of chlordiazepoxide during the first 24 hours.

CIWA – Ar Score	Frequency of subsequent observations		Administration of chlordiazepoxide
	Before first dose of chlordiazepoxide	After first and subsequent doses of chlordiazepoxide	
0-10	1 hourly	4 hourly	Nil
11-15	Half-hourly	2 hourly	Nil
16-20	2 hourly		25-50 mg
>20	2 hourly		50mg-75mg

NB. Maximum dose of chlordiazepoxide in first 24 hours should be 250mg unless advised otherwise by a Consultant or Senior Registrar.

Vitamin Supplementation

Parenteral vitamin supplements should be prescribed prophylactically for <u>all</u> in-patient detoxifications. There is considerable doubt about the usefulness of oral replacement.

Parenteral vitamin supplements should only be administered where suitable resuscitation facilities are available. The intramuscular route is usually used. Intravenous administration should be by dilution in 50-100 ml normal saline and infused over 15-30 minutes. This allows immediate discontinuation should anaphylaxis occur. Anaphylaxis is extremely rare after IM administration and this is the preferred route in most centres.

The classical triad of ophthalmoplegia, ataxia and confusion is rarely present in Wernicke's encephalopathy and the syndrome is much more common than is widely believed. A presumptive diagnosis of Wernicke's encephalopathy should therefore be made in any patient undergoing detoxification who experiences any of the following signs:

Ataxia	Hypothermia & hypotension
Confusion	Ophthalmoplegia/Nystagmus
Memory disturbance	Coma/Unconsciousness

Parenteral B-complex must be administered before glucose is administered in all patients presenting with altered mental status.

Prophylactic treatment for Wernicke's encephalopathy should be:

One pair IM/IV ampoules high potency B-complex vitamins (Pabrinex) daily for 3-5 days.

NB. All patients should receive this regimen as an absolute minimum.

Therapeutic treatment of Wernicke's encephalopathy should be:

At least two pairs IM/IV ampoules high potency B-complex vitamins daily for two days.

◆	No response, then discontinue treatment.

◆	If signs/symptoms respond, continue 1 pair ampoules daily for five days or for as long as improvement continues.

For out-patient detoxification, the options available are:

◆	No vitamin supplementation.

◆	Oral vitamin supplementation with vitamin B Compound Strong, one tablet three times daily (but this is unlikely to be absorbed effectively and therefore is of little or no benefit for most alcohol dependent patients).
◆	Parenteral supplementation, as above, in a clinic where appropriate resuscitation facilities are available.

Prescribing for Opioid Dependence

These guidelines are intended to provide information on the short-term management of patients presenting with opioid dependence. Long-term management should involve referral or contact with specialist services for advice.

Evidence of opioid dependence

Patient's self-reporting of opioid dependence must be confirmed by positive urine results for opioids, and objective signs of withdrawal or general restlessness should be present before considering to prescribe any substitute pharmacotherapy. Recent sites of injection may also be present.

Treatment Aims

✦ To reduce or prevent withdrawal symptoms.

✦ To stabilise drug intake and lifestyle.

✦ To reduce drug related harm (particularly injecting behaviour).

✦ To help maintain contact and provide an opportunity to work with the patient.

Treatment considerations

This will depend upon,

❖ What is available.

❖ Patient's previous history.

❖ Patient's current drug use and circumstances.

Substitute prescribing of Methadone

Methadone is a controlled drug with a high dependency potential and a low lethal dose. Prescribing should only commence if;

◆ Opioid drugs are being taken regularly (typically daily).

◆ There is convincing evidence of dependence (see above).

◆ Consumption of methadone can be supervised, especially for the initial doses.

Supervised daily consumption is recommended for new prescriptions, for a minimum of three months, if possible. Alternatively, installment prescriptions for daily dispensing and collection should be used. Certainly no more than one week's supply should be dispensed at one time, except in exceptional circumstances.

Methadone should be prescribed in the oral liquid formulation (mixture or linctus). Tablets are likely to be crushed and inappropriately injected, and therefore should not prescribed.

> Important: All patients starting a methadone treatment programme must be informed of the risks of toxicity and overdose, and the necessity for safe storage.

Dose

For patients who are currently prescribed methadone and if ALL the criteria listed below are met, then it is safe to prescribe the **same dose**.

❖ Dose confirmed by prescriber.

❖ Last consumption confirmed (eg.pharmacy contacted) and is within last three days.

❖ Prescriber has stopped prescribing, and current prescription is completed or cancelled to date.

❖ Patient is comfortable on dose (no signs of intoxication/withdrawal).

❖ No other contraindications or cautions are present.

Otherwise the following recommendations should be followed.

Starting Dose

Consideration must be given to the potential for opioid toxicity, taking into account:

◇ Patient's tolerance, which should be assessed on the history of quantity, frequency and route of administration (be aware of the likelihood of over reporting). A person's tolerance to methadone can be affected within 3-4 days of not using, caution must be exercised when re-instating their dose.

◇ Use of other drugs, particularly depressants e.g. alcohol and benzodiazepines.

◇ Long half-life of methadone, as cumulative toxicity may develop.

Inappropriate dosing can result in overdosing, particularly in the first few days. This can be fatal and deaths have occurred following the commencement of a daily dose of 40mg methadone. It is safer to keep to a low dose that can subsequently be increased at intervals, if proving to be insufficient.

Direct conversion tables for opioids and methadone should be viewed cautiously, as there are a number of factors influencing the values at any given time. It is much safer to titrate the dose against presenting withdrawal symptoms.

The initial daily dose for most cases will be in the range of 10-40mg methadone, depending on the level of tolerance (low; 10-20mg, moderate; 25-40mg). Starting doses greater than 30mg should be prescribed with caution, because of the risk of overdose. It is safer to use a starting dose of 10-20mg and re-assess the patient after a period of 4 hours. Further incremental doses of 5-10mg can be given, depending on the severity of the withdrawal symptoms.

Note: onset of action should occur within half an hour, with peak plasma levels being achieved after approximately 4 hours of dosing.

Heavily dependent users with high tolerance may require larger doses. A starting dose, not exceeding 40mg, can be given, followed by a second dose after a minimum interval of 4 hours. The second dose can be up to 30mg, depending on the persisting severity of withdrawal symptoms. Such doses should only be prescribed by experienced medical practitioners.

Severity of Withdrawal	Additional Dosage
Mild	Nil
Moderate (muscle aches & pains, pupil dilation, nausea, yawning)	5-10mg
Severe (vomiting, piloerection, tachycardia, elevated BP)	20-30mg

Stabilisation Dose

❑   First Week:
Out-patients should attend daily for the first few days to enable assessment by the prescriber and any dose titration against withdrawal symptoms. Dose increases should not exceed 5-10mg a day and 30mg a week, above the initial starting dose. Steady state plasma levels should be achieved five days after the last dose increase.

❑   Subsequent period:
Subsequent increases should not exceed 10mg per week, up to a total daily dose of 60-120mg. Stabilisation is usually achieved within six weeks but may take longer.

Cautions

❑   Intoxication. Methadone should not be given to any patient showing signs of intoxication, especially due to alcohol or other depressant drugs e.g. benzodiazepines. Risk of fatal overdose is greatly enhanced when methadone is taken concomitantly with alcohol and other respiratory depressant drugs. Concurrent alcohol and illicit drug consumption must be borne in mind when considering subsequent prescribing of methadone.

❑   Severe hepatic/renal dysfunction. Metabolism of methadone may be affected with lower doses required. The interval between assessments during initial dosing may need to be extended.

Overdose

In the case of methadone overdose naloxone should be administered, if available.

Dose: by intravenous injection, 0.8-2mg repeated at intervals of 2-3 minutes to a max. of 10mg if respiratory function does not improve.

If intravenous route not feasible, same dose can be given by intramuscular or subcutaneous injection, however onset of action may be slower.

By continuous intravenous infusion, 2mg diluted in 500ml intravenous infusion solution at a rate adjusted according to response.

Call Emergency Services.

Pregnancy & Breast Feeding

There is no evidence of an increase in congenital defects.

It is important to avoid the patient going into a withdrawal state. Specialist advice should be obtained before prescribing, particularly with regards to management and treatment plan during pregnancy.

Methadone is considered compatible with breast-feeding, with no adverse effects to nursing infant when mother is consuming 20mg/24hours or less.

Analgesia for Methadone prescribed patients

Non opioid analgesics should be used in preference, e.g. paracetamol, NSAIDs.

If opioid analgesia is indicated, e.g. codeine, dihydrocodeine, MST, then this should be titrated accordingly against pain relief, with the methadone dose remaining constant to alleviate withdrawal symptoms. Avoid titrating the methadone dose to provide analgesia.

Iofexidine

If substitute prescribing is not optional or desirable (e.g. patients with low dependence and/or tolerance), iofexidine can be used in the management of symptoms of opioid withdrawal.

Dose: initially, 200 micrograms twice daily, increased as necessary in steps of 200-400 micrograms daily to a max. 2.4mg daily.

Duration: 7-10 days, then withdraw gradually over 2-4 days.

Note: patients may require supplementary symptomatic treatment for nausea / vomiting, diarrhoea, and insomnia, during the first few days.

Objective scale – Clinician assessed

Objectives	Absent / Normal	Mild – Moderate	Severe
Lactorrhoea	absent	eyes watery	eyes streaming / wiping eyes
Rhinorrhoea	absent	sniffing	profuse secretion (wiping nose)
Agitation	absent	fidgeting	can't remain seated
Perspiration	absent	clammy skin	beads of sweat
Piloerection	absent	barely palpable hairs standing up	readily palpable, visible
Pulse rate (BPM)	< 80	≥80 but <100	≥100
Vomiting	absent	absent	present
Shivering	absent	absent	present
Yawning /10min	< 3	3-5	6 or more
Mydriasis	normal ≤4mm	dilated 4-6mm	widely dilated >6mm

Subjective scale – Patient reported

Subjectives	Absent	Mild	Moderate	Severe
Feeling sick				
Stomach cramps				
Muscle spasms/twitching				
Feelings of coldness				
Heart pounding				
Muscular tension				
Aches and pains				
Runny eyes				
Sweating				
Yawning				
Insomnia				

II) Alzheimer's Disease and Dementia

Drug Treatment of Alzheimer's Disease

Pathophysiology

✳ Destruction of cholinergic neurones, particularly in the cortex and hippocampus, is at least partly responsible for symptoms of Alzheimer's disease.

✳ Deficits in concentrations of choline acetyltransferase and acetylcholine have been observed and correlate with neuronal loss.

✳ Deficits in other neurotransmitters also occur.

✳ Destruction of neurones may be provoked by release of cytotoxic substances from microglial cells (e.g. following an ischaemic insult).

Mode of action

✳ Most drugs inhibit acetylcholinesterase and so prolong the activity of acetylcholine in the synapse.

✳ Some drugs are selective for acetylcholinesterase over butyrylcholinesterase. The latter is the soluble form of the enzyme found mainly in cardiac and smooth muscle. Inhibition of butyryl-cholinesterase is not necessary for efficacy but may increase adverse effects.

✳ Some drugs may inhibit release of cytotoxic compounds from microglial cells.

✳ Other modes of action are possible.

Drug activity

Alzeimer's drugs may be shown to be effective in the following areas:

Global	Behavioural and neuropsychiatric
Cognitive	Effect on burden to caregiver
Functional	Disease modification

Drugs usually provide overall slowing of deterioration in these areas, although improvement may be seen early in treatment. There is considerable individual variation in response. No drug has been shown unequivocally to modify disease progression.

Summary of Drug Properties in Alzheimer's Disease

Drug	Mode of action	Efficacy in:					Tolerability
		Global	Cognitive	Functional	Caregiver burden	Behavioural & neuro-psychiatric	
Tacrine	Acetylcholinesterase inhibitor	+	+	?	?	?	–
Donepezil	Acetylcholinesterase inhibitor	+	+	+	?	?	++[1]
Rivastigmine	Acetylcholinesterase inhibitor	+	+	+	?	?	++[1]
Metrifonate	Acetylcholinesterase inhibitor	+	+	+	+	+	+++(?)[2]
Propentofylline	Adenosine re-uptake inhibitor. Phosphodiesterase inhibitor	+	+	?	?	+(?)	?

KEY:
- – poor
- + moderate
- ++ good
- ? evidence absent/equivocal
- +++ very good

1. Tolerability dependent on dose and speed of titration.
2. Few reports of withdrawals due to adverse effects but some suggestions of more serious toxicity.

Drug Treatment of Alzheimer's disease – generic protocol

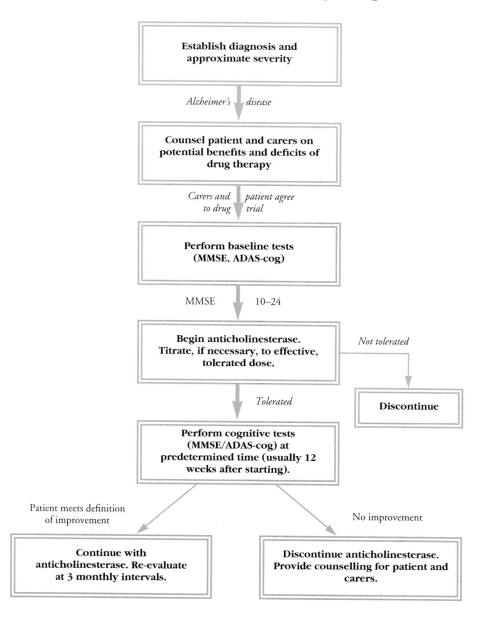

Establish diagnosis and approximate severity

Alzheimer's disease

Counsel patient and carers on potential benefits and deficits of drug therapy

Carers and patient agree to drug trial

Perform baseline tests (MMSE, ADAS-cog)

MMSE 10–24

Begin anticholinesterase. Titrate, if necessary, to effective, tolerated dose.

Not tolerated

Tolerated

Discontinue

Perform cognitive tests (MMSE/ADAS-cog) at predetermined time (usually 12 weeks after starting).

Patient meets definition of improvement

No improvement

Continue with anticholinesterase. Re-evaluate at 3 monthly intervals.

Discontinue anticholinesterase. Provide counselling for patient and carers.

Notes on Protocol for Drug Treatment of Alzheimer's Disease

❖ Diagnosis is best performed by a specialist, as are cognitive and functional tests.

❖ Counselling should include mention of the magnitude of effect likely, the possibility of adverse effects, and the likelihood of treatment failure.

❖ Commonly used cognitive tests include the Mini-Mental State Examination (MMSE) and the Alzheimer's Disease Assessment Scale – cognitive sub-scale (ADAS-cog). Many consider ADAS-cog unsuitable for routine clinical use. A number of other scales can be used.

❖ Anticholinesterase drugs have only been shown to be effective in patients with mild to moderate illness – usually a MMSE score of 10-24.

❖ Adverse effects include nausea, vomiting and diarrhoea. These effects are usually worse at higher doses and during rapid titration.

❖ "Improvement" is usually defined, somewhat arbitrarily, as a "worthwhile" change in MMSE and/or ADAS-cog. Exact values need to be defined locally, but are usually around 3 points on MMSE or -4 to -5 points on ADAS-cog at 3 months.

❖ Patients not meeting pre-determined criteria for improvement should be taken off drug therapy and provided with withdrawal counselling (include carers in this).

❖ Patients continuing after the first treatment evaluation are assumed to be "responders" and may continue with close monitoring. Note that deterioration is expected even in these responders and the decision to discontinue at some point must be taken on an individual basis.

❖ All drugs with anticholinergic effects should be avoided. Anticholinergic drugs may reduce the effect of anticholinesterases in all domains of efficacy: memory, activity, care-giver burden and behaviour may all be worsened.

Drugs to avoid:

Antipsychotics
–Chlorpromazine
–Clozapine
–Olanzapine
–Promazine
–Thioridazine

Antidepressants
–Tricyclic antidepressants
–Paroxetine
–MAOIs

Anticholinergics
–Benzhexol
–Benztropine
–Hyoscine
–Orphenadrine
–Procyclidine

III) Epilepsy

Treatment of Psychiatric Co-morbidity in People with Epilepsy (PWE)

General Recommendations for the use of Antiepileptic Drugs (AEDs)

● Choice of antiepileptic drugs (AEDs) should be made after considering the individual's epilepsy syndrome.

● Adverse psychotropic effects may be seen with all AEDs, but, of the standard AEDs, are particularly common with phenobarbitone and primidone. Phenytoin may also have both positive and negative psychotropic effects and the clinician must be aware of its high protein binding, inter-actions, and non-linear kinetics in prescribing. Consider changing to carbamazepine or valproate, if clinically appropriate. Clobazam is generally better tolerated than 1,4 benzodiazepines and may be an effective adjunct, although tolerance develops in some 50% of patients. It is also effective as an anxiolytic, although this represents an off-licence use. Its use is restricted to treatment of epilepsy.

● The data with respect to the psychotropic effects of the newer AEDs are inconclusive, but lam-otrigine and gabapentin may have some beneficial effects. Gabapentin has the advantage of very few drug interactions. Topiramate may cause adverse cognitive effects and must be titrated very slowly, over a period of months. Use of vigabatrin is severely limited because of neuropsychiatric toxicity and visual field defects and so BMJ guidelines should be followed if used. The extent of neuro-psychiatric side effects and visual field defects with tiagabine has not yet been elucidated.

● It is useful to monitor total plasma concentrations of the older AEDs; the clinical role of plasma monitoring with the newer AEDs is yet to be established. Free AED levels in patients on phenytoin and sodium valproate are also useful, particularly if other protein-bound agents are being used concurrently.

● Consider the possible contribution of folate deficiency related to AED therapy to an indi-vidual's psychiatric presentation; RBC folate levels should be screened.

● Avoid polytherapy.

● Modified release preparations of carbamazepine and valproate are probably better tolerated and need to be taken less frequently.

● Pre-conception counselling is essential for women of child-bearing age.

Psychiatric Co-morbidity in People with Epilepsy (PWE)

General Recommendations for the use of Psychotropics

● It is important to start psychotropics at a low dose and then to increase slowly. Most seizures occur after a dose increase.

● Treat with the lowest effective dose and review regularly.

● All non-MAOI antidepressants may lower seizure threshold. SSRIs appear to do so less than TCAs but more data are needed. Fluoxetine has the advantage of being the best studied, but may increase AED levels - at times precipitously. Trazodone, citalopram and sertraline have the advantage of fewer drug interactions, although increases in AED levels may still occur and levels should be monitored. There are few data with respect to moclobemide, but it appears to be safe in epilepsy. Of the TCAs, there is some evidence that doxepin may be less epileptogenic than others and clomipramine more epileptogenic. Maprotiline, amoxapine and bupropion should be avoided. The use of MAOIs (except moclobemide) is not recommended when the patient is on carbamazepine therapy.

● ECT may increase seizure threshold. If clinically indicated, ECT is a reasonable alternative to consider in people with epilepsy. Other nonpharmacological treatments should also be considered.

● All antipsychotics may lower the seizure threshold. Of the newer antipsychotics, clozapine and zotepine should particularly be avoided. Haloperidol and fluphenazine may be less epileptogenic and chlorpromazine more epileptogenic than other standard antipsychotics. There are few data available on the effect of newer antipsychotics on seizure threshold, but risperidone and sulpiride appear to be well tolerated and have the advantage of fewer extrapyramidal adverse effects in patients who require long-term treatment.

● Consider drug interactions. Psychotropics may increase anticonvulsant plasma levels and anticonvulsants may lower psychotropic plasma levels. Monitor anticonvulsant plasma levels closely.

● Certain populations may be more susceptible to the epileptogenic potential of psychotropics and this should be taken into account when treating the elderly, people with mental disability or a history of head trauma, alcohol or drug abuse and those withdrawing from benzodiazepines or barbiturates.

Treatment of Depression and Psychosis in Epilepsy
(Modified from McConnell and Duncan, 1998b)

Psychiatric Presentation	Treatment
Peri-ictal Depression	May be ictal or post-ictal affective symptoms; Inpatient admission for safety; Avoid antidepressants; Treat with optimisation of AEDs
Interictal Depression	Moclobemide, SSRIs (fluoxetine, sertraline); Consider citalopram and trazodone; Consider ECT; Avoid maprotiline, amoxapine, mianserin, clomipramine; Consider role of AED adverse effects; Consider stigma, psychosocial issues, suicide risk; Avoid phenobarbitone, primidone, vigabatrin; Cognitive therapy and insight-oriented psychotherapy are useful
Bipolar Disorder	Carbamazepine, sodium valproate Avoid phenobarbitone, primidone, vigabatrin; Consider ECT, lamotrigine, gabapentin Lithium is not contraindicated
Peri-ictal Psychosis	Decide whether symptoms are ictal or post-ictal and treat accordingly; If ictal, avoid antipsychotics; Ictal psychosis needs to be treated urgently; Consider short-term haloperidol in post-ictal psychosis; Treat with optimisation of AEDs; Inpatient admission for safety
Interictal Psychosis	Haloperidol, risperidone, sulpiride; Avoid clozapine, chlorpromazine and zotepine; Consider role of AED adverse effects; Avoid vigabatrin; Community support is important
Depression or Psychosis related to AED therapy	Short-term psychotropics only as above; Withdraw offending agent and substitute with appropriate AED; Check folate and B12 levels

Treatment of Anxiety Disorders in Epilepsy

(Modified from McConnell and Duncan, 1998b)

Psychiatric Presentation	Treatment
Anxiety/ Agoraphobia related to Locus of Control Issues	Cognitive therapy; Exposure; Psychotherapy; Education Psychotropics not generally indicated; Consider issues of self-esteem, driving, public perception, stigma
Ictal panic/anxiety	Psychotropics not indicated; Best treated with optimisation of AED treatment; Consider clobazam
Generalised Anxiety Disorder	Propranolol; Avoid short-acting benzodiazepines; Consider clobazam, clonazepam, Avoid long-term benzodiazepines unless indicated for seizure control, Consider relaxation; biofeedback; cognitive therapy
Simple Phobia	Psychotropics generally not indicated; Exposure in vivo; Systematic desensitization; Consider role of locus of control issues
Social Phobia	Propranolol, MAOIs; Avoid long-term benzodiazepines unless indicated for seizure control; Anxiety management
Obsessive- Compulsive Disorder	Paroxetine, fluoxetine; Avoid clomipramine; Consider clonazepam, if indicated, as well as for seizure control Consider thought stopping, exposure in vivo, response prevention
Panic Disorder	Paroxetine, MAOIs, clonazepam, imipramine (low dose) Avoid long-term benzodiazepines unless indicated for seizure control; Cognitive therapy; Relaxation exercises

Treatment of Other Psychiatric Co-Morbidity in Epilepsy
(Modified from McConnell and Duncan, 1998b)

Psychiatric Presentation	Treatment
Anorexia/ Bulimia	Fluoxetine; Avoid clomipramine; Sodium valproate may be the preferred AED; Avoid topiramate (weight loss); Behavioural modification techniques; Insight-oriented psychotherapy
Sexual Dysfunction	Avoid tricyclics and SSRIs; Consider switching to AED less likely to cause sexual dysfunction (e.g. lamotrigine); Consider role of AED adverse effects; Avoid carbamazepine, phenytoin, phenobarbitone, primidone; Treat underlying aetiology; Masters and Johnson techniques, education, involvement of partner and marital therapy are all useful
Cognitive Dysfunction	Use AEDs with fewer cognitive effects (carbamazepine, lamotrigine); Treat underlying cause if possible; Treat concomitant depression, agitation; Consider role of AED adverse effects; Consider role of seizures, transient cognitive impairment (TCI); Avoid phenobarbitone, primidone, topiramate; Use of a diary as an aid to memory and involvement of family important; Milieu therapy can be helpful
Nonepileptic Seizure-like Events (NESLEs)	Treatment should be directed at underlying cause; Consider psychiatric, medical and neurological causes of NESLEs; Consider possibility of NESLEs coexisting with epileptic seizures; Biofeedback, cognitive behavioural therapy and psychotherapy are useful
Aggression	Carbamazepine; sodium valproate ? lithium; ? buspirone Consider role of AED adverse effects; Avoid phenobarbitone, primidone; Behaviour modification and cognitive therapy are useful; Treat underlying cause of aggression
Attention Deficit Disorder	Treat with appropriate AED therapy in the first instance; Dexamphetamine and methylphenidate may be used if necessary; Consider role of AED adverse effects; Consider role of seizures, transient cognitive impairment (TCI); Avoid phenobarbitone, primidone; Behaviour modification techniques, supportive psychotherapy, family therapy and involvement of the school are all important

Use of Standard Antiepileptic Drugs (AEDs)

(Modified from McConnell and Duncan, 1998a,b)

AED	Primary Indications	Advantages	Disadvantages
Carbamazepine	Adjunctive or first line therapy in partial and generalised epilepsy (excluding absence and myoclonus); Lennox-Gastaut syndrome	Highly effective, inexpensive, well established; A drug of first choice in partial and generalised tonic-clonic seizures; Serum monitoring useful; Also useful as a mood stabiliser and for treatment of various pain conditions	Sedation, hyponatraemia, diplopia, ataxia, bone marrow dyscrasias, rash, Stevens-Johnson syndrome; Autoinduction; Be aware of possible cardiac toxicity in the elderly; Often poorly tolerated on initiation of therapy (transient); Many drug interactions
Clobazam	Adjunctive therapy in partial and generalised epilepsy; may be useful for intermittent therapy, one-off prophylaxis and catamenial seizures	Anxiolytic effects may be useful in concomitant panic disorder and other anxiety states; Excellent add-on therapy in treatment resistant patients	Sedation, agitation, disinhibition, withdrawal symptoms; Tolerance develops in up to half of patients, which severely limits its use
Clonazepam	Adjunctive therapy in partial and generalised epilepsy (including myoclonus and absence); Lennox-Gastaut syndrome; Infantile spasm; Status epilepticus	Some anxiolytic effects; Useful in children with refractory seizures; Some mood stabilising properties	Sedation particularly common, cognitive adverse effects, hyperactivity, aggression, withdrawal symptoms, ataxia, leucopenia; Usefulness limited by sedative and CNS effects and by tolerance
Ethosuximide	First-line or adjunctive therapy in generalised absence seizures. First line use declining.	A drug of first choice in absence seizures; Well established; Less hepatic toxicity than valproate in children; Serum monitoring useful	Gastric upset, ataxia, sedation, diplopia, psychosis, behavioural disturbance, rash, blood dyscrasias; Only effective in absence seizures

Drug	Indications	Comments	Side effects
Phenobarbitone (PB) and Primidone (PMD)	Previously used as adjunctive or first line therapy in partial and generalised epilepsy (excluding absence and myoclonus); status epilepticus (PB)	Inexpensive, effective, well established; IV preparation available for treatment of status epilepticus (PB); Serum monitoring useful but complicated by tolerance	Sedation, ataxia, hyperkinesis and learning difficulties (children), aggression, cognitive and sexual dysfunction, folate, vitamin K and D deficiency, withdrawal seizures; Not recommended in people with psychiatric co-morbidity
Phenytoin	Adjunctive or first line therapy in partial and generalised epilepsy (excluding absence and myoclonus); status epilepticus	Inexpensive, effective, well established; IV preparation available for treatment of status epilepticus; Serum monitoring mandatory	Sedation, gingival hyperplasia, hirsutism, blood dyscrasias, folate and Vitamin K deficiency; hypersensitivity, ataxia, dyskinesias, hepatitis; Many drug interactions; Non-linear kinetics
Sodium Valproate	Adjunctive or first line therapy in partial and generalised epilepsy (including myoclonus and absence); Lennox-Gastaut syndrome; Juvenile myoclonic epilepsy	A drug of first choice in primary generalised epilepsies with the widest spectrum of efficacy of AEDs; Also effective as a mood stabiliser; Available as IV preparation	Weight gain, hair loss, severe hepatic toxicity in young children, blood dyscrasias, gastric upset, sedation, pancreatitis, tremor, hyperammonaemia; significant drug interaction with lamotrigine

Use of Newer Antiepileptic Drugs (AEDs)

The newer AEDs are being increasingly used for first and second line therapy in many epilepsies. For example, lamotrigine has found an important role in the treatment of juvenile myoclonic epilepsy and many primary generalised syndromes in addition to its other indications. Gabapentin is well tolerated and has few interactions. Although it is used routinely in doses well above 3g overseas, its maximum dose recommendation in the BNF remains at 2400 mg daily. Gabapentin is also used off-licence overseas for various pain states particularly diabetic neuropathy and other neuropathic pain syndromes. Both gabapentin and lamotrigine are used off-license as mood stabilisers. Topiramate initially developed problems with adverse effects related to its rapid titration which have been shown to improve somewhat with the slower schedule more recently introduced.

Concern over both the behavioural toxicity (particularly depression and psychosis) and the impairment in visual fields due to vigabatrin have caused many to reserve their use of this agent for very specific indications. It is still widely used in the UK for the treatment of infantile spasms and guidelines have recently been developed to assist the clinician in monitoring patients for the development of visual field defects and are available on the web for reference (www.bmj.com). The data are too few at this time to evaluate potential positive or negative behavioural side effects of tiagabine, launched in the UK in the later part of 1998. There have been reports of visual field loss occurring with tiagabine use within recent months. The patients with these problems were also taking a variety of other medications. The manufacturer points out that the evidence is not as strong as for vigabatrin in this regard and that a pilot study of 30 monotherapy patients on tiagabine is currently underway to evaluate the severity of this and to elucidate these preliminary findings (personal communication, Sanofi, December, 1998).

Other AEDs, which should be mentioned here, include piracetam, which is useful for cerebral myoclonus and well tolerated. It is touted on the internet for its so-called 'smart drug' effects, but there is only anecdotal evidence as to its cognitive effects at present. Its sister drug levetiracetam appears effective for other types of seizures and is also well tolerated at this stage but has not yet been approved for use. Fos-phenytoin, a new parenteral preparation of phenytoin, has just been approved for use in the UK and has the advantage of being able to be administered intramuscularly and to be safer and better tolerated than the previous preparations of parenteral phenytoin. Its role for the psychiatrist seeing patients with epilepsy remains to be elucidated but it appears very promising as an agent of choice for the treatment of status epilepticus in a psychiatric setting.

The guidelines presented here are meant to reflect the use of these agents in a psychiatric setting i.e. in the presence of psychiatric co-morbidity. The reader is referred to the guidelines of the Royal College of Physicians and the Institute of Neurology for treatment of adults with refractory epilepsy and to those of the Scottish Intercollegiate Guideline Network for treatment of seizures in a general neurology or medical setting.

Use of Newer Antiepileptic Drugs (AEDs)

Modified from McConnel and Duncan (1998a,b)

AED	Primary Indications	Advantages	Disadvantages
Fosphenytoin	Status epilepticus	Parenteral formulation which can be given IM or IV; Better tolerated than older IV phenytoin parenteral preparations (less cardiac toxicity)	Probably has similar behavioural effect profile to phenytoin, but its exact role in a psychiatric setting remains to be elucidated
Gabapentin	Adjunctive therapy in refractory partial and secondarily generalised epilepsy; seizures occurring in porphyria	Few drug interactions; well tolerated; may be particularly useful in patients on multiple drugs or with hepatic impairment; may be titrated more quickly than other new AEDs; ? mood stabilising effects; effective in some pain states	Drowsiness, ataxia and nausea at high doses; seizure exacerbation reported; several case reports of behavioural disturbance in children with severe learning disabilities
Lamotrigine	Adjunctive or monotherapy in partial and generalised epilepsy; Lennox–Gastaut syndrome; Juvenile myoclonic epilepsy	Effective and well tolerated; few adverse behavioural or cognitive effects; wide spectrum of efficacy; may have some mood stabilising effects	Rash (may be severe). Serious rash more common in children; headache, ataxia, nausea, insomnia; Autoinduction; Drug interactions especially with standard AEDs
Piracetam	Cerebral myoclonus	Well tolerated; ? beneficial cognitive effects	Needs to be taken in large doses to be effective
Tiagabine	Add-on treatment of partial seizures with and without secondary generalisation	Few drug interactions; ? anxiolytic effects; ? usefulness in tardive dyskinesia	Dizziness, blurred vision, headache, rash, ? depression, ?psychosis; ? visual field effects
Topiramate	Adjunctive therapy in refractory partial and secondarily generalised epilepsy	Highly effective	Cognitive dysfunction, confusion, agitation, weight loss, dizziness, tremor, depression, renal calculi; Drug interactions with phenytoin and carbamazepine; Must be titrated slowly; Use limited by CNS toxicity
Vigabatrin	Adjunctive therapy in refractory partial and secondarily generalised epilepsy; Lennox–Gastaut syndrome; infantile spasms	Highly effective new AED for infantile spasms; Very few drug interactions	Sedation, dizziness, aggression, depression, psychosis, weight gain, ataxia, diarrhoea, case reports of irreversible peripheral field defects; Use severely limited by neuropsychiatric toxicity and by visual field deficits; Guidelines for monitoring of visual fields published by the BMJ (vol 317, p 1322) should be followed

Important Interactions of Antiepileptic Drugs (AEDs) in Psychiatry

(Modified from McConnell and Duncan, 1998b)

AED	Psychotropic Interactions	Effects on Other AEDs	Other Interactions
Carbamazepine	CBZ may decrease levels of: antipsychotics (clozapine, haloperidol), TCAs, paroxetine, BZDs; CBZ levels may be increased by: viloxazine, TCAs, SSRIs; Presumed enhanced bone marrow toxicity with CBZ and clozapine; Increased risk of serotonin syndrome with SSRIs (case report); Theoretical increased risk of hypertensive crisis with MAOIs	Increased metabolism of PHT: will usually decrease, but may increase plasma levels of PHT; Decreased plasma levels of lamotrigine, tiagabine, topiramate and valproate; May decrease plasma levels of ethosuximide and primidone (by increased conversion to PHB)	Dextropropoxyphene, tramadol, erythromycin, isoniazid, warfarin, calcium channel blockers, lithium, danazol, corticosteroids, cyclosporin, diuretics, oral contraceptives, theophylline, thyroxine, paracetamol, cimetidine, vitamin D
Ethosuximide	None known	May increase plasma levels of PHT	Isoniazid, ? oral contraceptives
Gabapentin	None known	No known interactions with other AEDs; Isolated report of interaction with PHT	None known
Lamotrigine	None known	Case reports of increased plasma levels of 10-11, epoxide (CBZ metabolite), and of valproate	Paracetamol
Phenobarbitone	PHB may decrease levels of: antipsychotics, TCAs, paroxetine, BZDs; Additive sedative effects with antipsychotics, TCAs and BZDs; SSRIs may increase PHB levels; MAOIs may decrease PHB metabolism	Increased metabolism and decreased half-life of PHT, will usually decrease but may increase plasma levels of PHT; Decreased plasma levels of CBZ, clonazepam, lamotrigine, tiagabine and valproate; May decrease plasma levels of ethosuximide	Alcohol, disopyramide, warfarin, antibiotics, calcium channel blockers, thyroxine, corticosteroids, paracetamol, cyclosporin, theophylline, oral contraceptives, vitamin D

Phenytoin	PHT may decrease levels of: antipsychotics (clozapine), TCAs, paroxetine, BZDs; Phenothiazines may increase or decrease PHT levels; PHT levels may be increased by: TCAs, SSRIs; BZDs may increase or decrease PHT levels; Additive sedation with BZDs	Decreased half-life of PHB, increased or decreased plasma levels of PHB; Increased metabolism of BZDs, and increased clearance; Decreased plasma levels of lamotrigine, tiagabine, topiramate and valproate; Increased or decreased plasma levels of CBZ; Decreased plasma levels of ethosuximide and primidone (by increased conversion to PHB)	Aspirin, antacids, amiodarone, quinidine, disopyramide, mexiletine, antibiotics, warfarin, tolbutamide, antifungals, antimalarials, zidovudine, calcium channel blockers, corticosteroids, cyclosporin, methotrexate, disulfiram, carbonic anhydrase inhibitors, enteral foods, lithium, oral contraceptives, folate, theophylline, thyroxine, cimetidine, sucralfate, paracetamol, omeprazole, sulphinpyrazone, influenza vaccine, vitamin D
Tiagabine	Nefazodone and fluoxetine may increase tiagabine levels	May cause minor (10%) decreases in valproate levels	As tiagabine is metabolised by CYP3A4, erythromycin, grapefruit juice, and ketoconozole may increase tiagabine's plasma levels and rifampicin may reduce them
Topiramate	None known	May increase plasma levels of PHT	Oral contraceptives
Valproate	Case report of hepatotoxicity (chlorpromazine); SSRIs may increase valproate levels (case reports); Valproate may increase BZD levels; Increased and decreased clozapine levels reported	Increased PHB and lamotrigine levels; May decrease plasma levels of CBZ; May increase 10, 11 epoxide levels (CBZ metabolite); Increased or decreased plasma levels of PHT; May increase plasma levels of ethosuximide and primidone; May increase free tiagabine concentrations	Aspirin, cholestyramine, antimalarials, cimetidine
Vigabatrin	None known	Decreased plasma levels of PHT; May decrease plasma levels of PHB and primidone	None known

Abbreviations: SSRIs = selective serotonin reuptake inhibitors; TCAs = tricyclic antidepressants; MAOIs= monoamine oxidase inhibitors; BZD= benzodiazepines; PHB= phenobarbitone; CBZ= carbamazepine; PHT= phenytoin; AED= antiepileptic drugs
Note benzodiazepine interactions are listed under the psychotropic interaction column.

IV) Gilles de la Tourette's Syndrome

❖ Gilles de la Tourette's syndrome (GTS) is characterised by the occurrence of motor and vocal tics and is usually of childhood onset. *Psychiatric co-morbidity* is common and may take a variety of forms. GTS is most frequently associated with obsessive-compulsive disorder (OCD), but may also be associated with other anxiety disorders, depression, and attention deficit disorder with hyperactivity (ADHD). Apart from a few case reports, there is no clear association of GTS with psychosis. The psychological and psychosocial reactions to this chronic neurological illness must also be considered in the treatment of GTS.

❖ The decision about whether to treat and, if so, what type of treatment to use, will depend on the degree to which the tics are interfering with the patient's ability to function productively.

❖ Start patients on the smallest dose of medication that is possible.

❖ Increase the dosage gradually paying close attention to the development of side effects as well as diminution of symptoms.

❖ Assure an adequate duration of any drug trial on sufficient dosage.

❖ Make changes in regimens slowly as sequences of single steps.

❖ When discontinuing medication be careful not to confuse withdrawal reactions with a need for more medication.

❖ Small doses of haloperidol (0.25-0.5 mg daily increasing by weekly intervals of 0.5 mg; usual maintenance dose: 2-3 mg) are useful in treating the *motor and vocal tics* associated with GTS. However, extrapyramidal symptoms, sedation and tardive dyskinesia are particular concerns with its use in this population. Sulpiride has fewer EPS, perhaps including tardive dyskinesia, and sedative effects and may be better tolerated by many. Gynaecomastia, galactorrhoea and menstrual problems have been reported with its use. Other antipsychotics may also be effective for treatment of tics, particularly fluphenazine and risperidone. Clonidine has the advantage of being well tolerated with no EPS and may be useful on its own or in augmenting the effects of antipsychotics. Small doses of pimozide are also effective in treating the tics in GTS, but its use requires ECG monitoring because of its cardiac effects. Dronabinol and other THC derivatives have been reported anecdotally to be of symptomatic assistance in GTS, but are not licensed in the UK for medical purposes.

❖ If *obsessive compulsive disorder* (OCD) is present, SSRIs are the treatment of choice. Currently only fluoxetine, paroxetine and fluvoxamine are licensed for use in OCD. Clomipramine is also effective but is less well tolerated. The use of buspirone for anxiety symptoms may increase motor tics. These same choices of antidepressants are useful in the treatment of *depression* in this population, as there are frequently obsessive-compulsive symptoms that are associated with the depressive illness. Other SSRIs or tricyclics may also be used safely. Behavioural therapy may be a useful adjunctive treatment.

❖ Clonidine is the treatment of choice if *ADHD* is present, as it may be effective in treating both the tics and the behavioural symptoms. Imipramine has been reported effective in this population as well and is preferable to the use of stimulants which may cause additional dykinesias. Methylphenidate and amphetamines are both effective in the treatment of ADHD, but regular monitoring for stimulant-induced dyskinesias is advised. Behavioural therapies are also very important in the treatment of ADHD in GTS.

Condition	Treatment Recommendations
Motor and Vocal Tics	Clonidine Haloperidol Pimozide* Sulpiride
Obsessive Compulsive Disorder	Clomipramine SSRIs (fluoxetine, paroxetine, fluvoxamine)
Attention Deficit Hyperactivity Disorder (ADHD)	Clonidine Dexamphetamine Imipramine Methylphenidate
Depression	Clomipramine SSRIs

* **low dose only; ECG monitoring required**

132

V) Head Trauma And Acquired Brain Injury (ABI)

General Principles

◆ ABI can present with a variety of psychiatric symptoms

◆ Complex partial seizures can produce a wide range of behavioural manifestations

◆ Patients are often on other medical and CNS active drugs; beware of interactions.

◆ Avoid prn medication (variable blood levels; may reinforce unwanted behaviours).

◆ Adverse effects from psychotropics are more common after ABI, particularly drug-induced akathisia, increased sensitivity to anticholinergic effects, decreased seizure threshold, increased propensity to sedation and confusion.

◆ Depression may be as common as 50% post ABI. The best predictor of depression is a previous history of depression. Always consider when deterioration is noted, particularly in early post-ABI recovery.

◆ Mania can be difficult to distinguish from early post ABI agitation until symptoms become more clearly defined. It may occur as a one-off episode in the absence of a previous history; an attempt to taper medication after the first episode should be considered.

◆ Dyscontrol and disinhibition are common and sometimes associated with orbital frontal and anterior temporal damage.

◆ Consider akathisia in the differential diagnosis of aggression, irritability or agitation in this population because of their susceptibility to this adverse effect

◆ There are many factors contributing to the genesis of psychiatric comorbidity following head injury, including: premorbid personality, emotional impact of injury, circumstances of injury, repercussions of injury, iatrogenic factors, compensation issues, potential development of seizures, amount and location of injury (after Lishman, 1998).

◆ The degree and length of post-traumatic amnesia (PTA) relates to the development of psychiatric disability and intellectual impairment.

◆ If the PTA exceeds 24 hours, the likelihood of significant intellectual impairment increases markedly.

◆ Cognitive impairment, personality change, psychosis (schizophrenia, paranoid, affective), neurosis, and the ill-defined "post-traumatic syndrome" are all reported to occur following traumatic brain injury.

◆ Rehabilitation of intellectual impairment should involve the confidence and full co-operation of the patient, an optimistic approach, a graded programme, and careful attention to physical and psychological health. Retraining in attentional mechanisms may be beneficial and detection and treatment of underlying depression is important.

♦ One cannot underestimate the role of social adaptation and the effects on the family of head injury. Expressed Emotion ('EE') can be an important factor in the prediction of relapse and should be considered in the treatment plan of patients with head injury.

♦ EE has been hypothesised (McConnell and Duncan, 1998b) to relate to the social apraxia that may develop as a result of the patient losing the ability to recognise facial emotions in others and important social cues, usually due to right-sided injury or lesions of the amygdala. The subsequent interactions with the family may relate to the genesis of EE and should be considered in the family therapy sessions as part of rehabilitation.

♦ Choice of psychotropics should include consideration of epileptogenicity, potential interactions with other medications and the increased risk of adverse effects.

♦ Psychotropic medication should be started at a low dose and increased slowly, according to efficacy and tolerability.

Treatment of Psychiatric Comorbidity Following Acquired Brain Injury

Condition	Recommended Treatment
Abulia	✦ Exclude other aetiologies e.g. depression, sedation from antipsychotics, negative symptoms of schizophrenia-like psychosis ✦ Behavioural interventions ✦ Dopamine agonists such as bromocriptine or lisuride may occasionally be helpful in the hands of a clinician experienced with their use
Bipolar Disorder	✦ Valproate or antipsychotics (haloperidol) may be useful in acute stages ✦ Carbamazepine and lithium, initiated gradually, may be used for prophylaxis, if indicated; however, episodes of mania/agitation can occur as isolated events and do not necessarily recur
Delirium	✦ General supportive care (consider metabolic causes, drugs or withdrawal syndromes as a cause of confusion) ✦ Short term sedation with clonazepam/chlormethiazole ✦ Consider risperidone or sulpiride if an antipsychotic is needed ✦ Carbamazepine and buspirone may also be considered
Depression	✦ Social support and multidisciplinary approach is very important; involving relatives where possible ✦ Cognitive and behavioural treatment should be used as adjunctive therapy ✦ SSRIs treatment of choice ✦ ECT to be avoided in first 6 months post injury
Dyscontrol / Disinhibition	✦ Exclude other psychiatric pathology/epilepsy ✦ Mainly behavioural assessments to identify triggers etc ✦ Drugs may be useful e.g. carbamazepine and beta blockers (Lewin & Sumners,1992; Greendyke et al, 1986) ✦ Benzodiazepines may worsen symptoms
Psychosis	✦ Most post ABI psychoses respond well to antipsychotic agents, but patients are more likely to suffer adverse effects ✦ Sulpiride may be drug of choice; best to use less epileptogenic antipsychotics (see section above) ✦ Assess response in the usual way after 6-8 week trial ✦ Carbamazepine has been reported to be effective in some cases
Social Apraxia	✦ Social apraxia has been hypothesised (McConnell and Duncan, 1998b) to be related to an inability to pick up social cues and to recognise facial emotions due usually to right-sided lesions and/or to damage to the amygdala ✦ Social apraxia often confused with personality issues, but important to recognise as represents a treatable cause of such behavioural and social problems ✦ Such a loss of ability to recognise facial features and key social cues is best approached from a practical, skill-based perspective using communication skills training, group therapy and anger management.

VI) Multiple Sclerosis

❖ *Depression* is a common occurrence in patients with multiple sclerosis (MS), occurring with a point prevalence of approximately 27%. Depression may be due to a psychological reaction to a chronic neurological illness, related to the illness itself or to treatment with beta interferon, ACTH or steroids. Pathological laughter and pathological crying may also occur and be independent of the underlying emotional state of the individual. *Apathy states* and *abulia* as well as disorders of *lability of affect* may occur. Personality changes, intellectual impairment and euphoria are also common in patients with MS. There are also some case reports of *psychosis* in MS. There are few data available to suggest *treatment strategies* in psychiatric co-morbidity in MS. Below are some general considerations for prescribing of psychotropics in this population.

❖ Tricyclics are effective in treating depression in this disorder, but are not well tolerated, with very high drop out rates related to anticholinergic effects. SSRIs are effective, at least in one retrospective study with sertraline, and appear to be well tolerated. Sertraline (and probably other SSRIs) are thus preferred as antidepressants of choice.

❖ If psychiatric effects are felt related to medical therapy of MS, treatment should be directed at removal or reduction in dosage of the causal agent. Beta–interferon has been associated with adverse psychiatric effects, particularly depression and lethargy. Side effects are generally dose related. Steroids and baclofen (for spasticity) have also been associated with depression and psychosis and neither are well tolerated in abrupt withdrawal.

❖ There are recent reports of cannabinoids being effective for 'well-being' and for analgesia in MS. There is currently, however, no licence for the medical use of this class of drugs in the UK.

❖ There are few data available as to choice of antipsychotics in MS. Drugs that have fewer EPS and anticholinergic effects (e.g. olanzapine, risperidone) may, however, be better tolerated in this population.

136

VII) Parkinson's Disease

❖ *Depression* is a common manifestation of Parkinson's disease (PD) occurring in about 1/3 of patients in the community and about 1/2 of hospital patients. The characteristic loss of facial expression, psychomotor retardation, alterations in gait and changes in speech, typical of early PD, should not be mistaken for a sign of depression, however, and a careful mental state examination should clarify the issue. Depression and anhedonia must be present to confirm the diagnosis of depression. Note that an amotivational syndrome occurs in one third of patients and this should be differentiated from depression. *Mania*, on the other hand, is rare in PD and is usually due to dopaminergic treatment when present.

❖ *Tricyclics* are effective in treating depression in PD and may also be helpful from the standpoint of EPS by virtue of their anticholinergic activity; however, tricyclics may also uncommonly cause EPS and may impair absorption of levodopa. The anticholinergic activity may also increase confusion in the elderly. Of the tricyclics, lofepramine has the advantage of fewer adverse cardiac effects and less serotonergic activity. Nortriptyline has been shown to be effective and well tolerated in one double-blind placebo-controlled study. Imipramine and desipramine (now discontinued) have also been found to be efficacious in treating depression in PD. Amoxapine should be avoided because of its potential to cause Pakinsonism.

❖ *SSRIs* may be effective in treating depression associated with PD, although there have been no controlled trials and there have been case reports of fluoxetine and paroxetine exacerbating the motor symptoms in PD. All SSRIs have tremor as a common adverse effect. SSRIs and clomipramine should not be used with selegiline as there are reports of serotonergic reactions as well as of increased EPS with this combination.

❖ *MAOIs* (including *moclobemide*) interact with levodopa, causing hypertensive crisis and should thus be avoided in PD. They also may interact with selegiline and this combination is also not recommended. If selegiline is used with moclobemide, full MAO inhibition may occur and full MAOI dietary precautions are necessary. Selegiline itself may have some antidepressant effects as well as effects on the movement disorder in PD.

❖ Of the *mood stabilising agents*, sodium valproate and lithium can both cause tremor independently of PD and this may be difficult to differentiate from the primary tremor associated with PD. Sodium valproate has also been associated with other EPS. Consider the possibility of these agents affecting the tremor in PD if it is exacerbated after starting them or increasing their dosage, even if serum levels are in the 'therapeutic' range. Carbamazepine is preferred as a mood stabiliser in PD.

❖ *Electroconvulsive therapy* (ECT) is a useful treatment for depression in PD and may also alleviate the parkinsonian symptoms, albeit temporarily.

❖ *Psychosis* occurs in 20-30% of patients. It is frequently caused by treatment of PD and its therapy should, in the first instance be directed at reducing or stopping the most recently added antiparkinsonian agent. Otherwise antiparkinsonian agents should be reduced or discontinued in the following order: anticholinergics, MAO-B inhibitors, amantadine, dopamine receptor agonists. If there is no improvement in psychotic symptoms, then levodopa should be gradually reduced. Administering levodopa after food intake may slow its absorption and diminish its adverse psychiatric effects. If there is still no improvement in symptoms, olanzapine or clozapine should be added with reassessment of motor status. If an aggravation of motor symptoms occurs, antiparkinsonian agents should be cautiously reintroduced in the reverse order given above.

❖ Avoid use of *antipsychotics* with a particularly high propensity to cause extrapyramidal side effects (EPS) e.g. haloperidol, phenothiazines. Consider the use of atypical antipsychotics which may have fewer EPS e.g. clozapine, olanzapine, sulpiride. Of these, clozapine has been most studied and may have some beneficial effects on the EPS of PD in addition to effectively treating the psychosis. It should be noted, however, that the elderly may be more predisposed to agranulocytosis with clozapine. Clozapine is also licensed only for the treatment of refractory schizophrenia and, as its prescribing is tightly controlled, it may be difficult to get approval for its use in a non-schizophrenic population. There are conflicting reports of the use of risperidone, with some reporting this to be effective and others reporting exacerbation of EPS with its use in PD. Olanzapine has been found effective and well tolerated in at least one small study and quetiapine has been used with good results in two patients. If a standard antipsychotic is used, thioridazine may be preferred as it has a lower incidence of EPS.

❖ *Dopamine dyskinesias* (DD) are very common in patients treated with long-term levodopa and may also occur after only 4 weeks of therapy. This must be differentiated from tardive dyskinesia in the case of patients treated with concomitant antipsychotics.

❖ *Dementia* occurs up to 10 times more frequently in patients with PD, depending on the particular parkinsonian syndrome. Aggressive treatment of depression and minimising the use of anticholinergics may help to reduce cognitive deficits. Conversely, cholinomimetic agents may be of benefit.

❖ *Anxiety* is also a common occurrence in PD. It occurs early in the course of PD and may be associated with a depressive illness. If benzodiazepines are used, it should be noted that they may occasionally antagonise the effects of levodopa.

Psychotropic Group	Recommendations
Antidepressants	Lofepramine Nortriptyline
Antipsychotics	Clozapine Olanzapine ? Quetiapine ? Sulpiride
Mood stabilisers	Carbamazepine

VIII) Porphyria

❖ The porphyrias are associated with a variety of neuropsychiatric manifestations, including seizures, psychosis and affective symptoms. They may be associated with abdominal pain and/or with a discolouration of urine during attacks, but these features may also be absent.

❖ There are many types of porphyrias and the diagnostic tests for evaluation and drugs which exacerbate each syndrome are different. Note also the difficulties inherent in diagnosing acute porphyria; obtaining bloods and urines during the acute symptomatic phase may be important.

❖ Acute porphyria may be exacerbated by many drugs and an acute exacerbation is treated with haemarginate. Vomiting can be treated with promazine and pain can be treated with pethidine, dihydrocodeine or morphine.

❖ Gabapentin and sodium valproate are the safer AEDs.

❖ Close attention to electrolytes may be important, particularly if vomiting is present. The following psychotropics are to be avoided in porphyria as they have been associated with precipitating acute attacks:

– *amphetamines*

– *tricyclic and related antidepressants (except amitriptyline and lofepramine)*

– *monoamine oxidase inhibitors (MAOIs)*　　– *carbamazepine*

– *benzodiazepines (?)*　　– *lamotrigine*

barbiturates　　– *phenytoin*

Advice on the safety of medical and psychiatric therapies in this disorder is available from the National Porphyria Service (01222 742979). The clinician is advised to telephone with concerns about both diagnosis and treatment before starting treatment in known or suspected porphyria as information about possible adverse effects is constantly changing. This Centre has produced a bulletin on this topic and have available a list of drugs which are considered safe in the acute porphyrias.

Psychotropic Group	Recommendations
Antidepressants	Amitriptyline Fluoxetine Lofepramine
Antipsychotics	Chlorpromazine Droperidol Haloperidol Trifluoperazine
Mood Stabilisers	Lithium Sodium valproate

IX) Stroke

❖ Depression is a common occurrence following a stroke, affecting approximately one third of patients. The greatest risk is within the first two years of a stroke and those with left - anterior or right - posterior lesions are at greater risk. Those with non-fluent aphasia are also at greater risk, although it is not clear whether this is a causal relationship or whether it is an independent outcome arising from damage in the same region. Left hemisphere lesions may also be related to the development of cognitive impairment with depression. Depression may relate to a psychological reaction to the illness and/or to the site of brain injury itself or nature and degree of disability. Other risk factors for the development of depression include a personal or family history of depression, and the presence of subcortical atrophy preceding the stroke.

❖ The choice of antidepressant following a stroke is dependent on the age of the patient, the potential for epileptogenicity of the lesion, the use of anticoagulant therapy or of other cardiac drugs, and the efficacy of the antidepressant in this population. Because many patients with cerebrovascular disease are also elderly and have concomitant cardiac disease, the recommendations set out in both these sections generally apply to this population as well. Consideration of the epileptogenic potential of psychotropics is also important, as the brain injury sustained as a result of the stroke puts the patient at an increased risk for development of seizures and an antidepressant with low epileptogenic potential is also preferred (see section on Epilepsy). As concerns efficacy, there are few data available, but studies have been done showing nortriptyline, citalopram and trazodone to be effective in treating post-stroke depression. Tricyclics, however, are often poorly tolerated in this population and their anticholinergic effects, adverse cardiac profile and epileptogenicity make them a less desirable choice for the treatment of post-stroke depression. SSRIs and moclobemide are thus the antidepressants of choice in this population.

❖ Drug interactions are an important consideration in the selection of psychotropics in this population. Many patients will be on aspirin which will increase the free plasma concentrations of highly protein-bound drugs (e.g. sodium valproate, fluoxetine, paroxetine, sertraline amongst others). Patients on anticoagulant therapy with warfarin (e.g. those at risk of embolic stroke, atrial fibrillation) present a particular problem in the choice of antidepressants because of potential interactions which may increase the INR and cause potentially serious haemhorragic complications. These are summarised in the following table.

❖ Citalopram may be less likely than nefazodone and sertraline to interact with warfarin. Fluoxetine and fluvoxamine appear to have the highest potential of the antidepressants for interactions. Interactions of other cardiac medications should also be considered.

Psychotropic interactions with warfarin

(Modified from Duncan et al, 1998 and Greenblatt et al, 1998)

Antidepressant	Mechanisms of Potential Interaction
SSRIs	Fluoxetine: Highly protein bound; moderate inhibitor of CYP2C9, CYP2C19 and CYP3A;? substrate at CYP2C9 Fluvoxamine: Not highly protein bound; potent inhibitor of CYP1A2 and CYP2C19; moderate inhibitor of CYP2C9 and CYP3A; ? substrate at CYP1A2 Paroxetine: Highly protein bound Sertraline: Highly protein bound; ? substrate at CYP2C9 and CYP3A; minor to moderate inhibitor of CYP2C19 Citalopram: Not highly protein bound; not a major inhibitor of isozymes; substrate at CYP2C19 and CYP3A
Nefazodone	Highly protein bound; potent inhibitor of CYP3A; substrate at CYP3A
Trazodone	Highly protein bound; Substrate at CYP1A2; P450 metabolism poorly understood; single case report
Venlafaxine	Not highly protein bound; substrate at CYP2C19 and CYP3A; no interaction studies available
Moclobemide	Not highly protein bound;? inhibitor of CYP1A2 and CYP2C19; substrate at CYP2C19; no interaction studies available
MAOIs (tranylcypromine)	May inhibit cytochrome P450 (inhibits CYP2C19); extent of protein binding is not known
TCAs	Highly protein bound; substrate at CYP1A2, CYP2C19, and/or CYP3A; anticholinergic effects may slow gastric motility and thus increase time available for dissolution and absorption of warfarin

❖ Pathological crying ('emotional incontinence', 'pseudobulbar affect') may occur after stroke and is, characteristically, unrelated to the inner emotional state of the individual. Nortriptyline, amitriptyline and citalopram have been shown to alleviate pathological crying after stroke.

❖ Post-stroke apathy may occur independently of depression following stroke and may be difficult to differentiate from an affective illness.

❖ Mania is a rare (<1%) manifestation of acute stroke and may occur more frequently in right orbitofrontal or basotemporal lesions or through diaschisis. There are no controlled trials of the treatment of bipolar disorder or of mania following stroke. Because of the epileptogenic potential of the lesion following stroke, however, sodium valproate and carbamazepine may be preferable to lithium in treating this population. If carbamazepine is used in patients with concomitant cardiac disease, a baseline ECG should be obtained as well as regular cardiac monitoring.

❖ *Post-stroke psychosis* is also relatively uncommon and may occur as part of a delirium or as an hallucinosis. The same considerations for the choice of antipsychotics apply as in the elderly and in patients with epilepsy and cardiac disease. Other psychiatric manifestations following stroke include generalised *anxiety* (often associated with depression), *anosognosia* (especially in right hemisphere lesions), and the so-called '*catastrophic reaction*' seen with anterior cortical lesions and, at times, with aphasia. A catastrophic reaction occurs in about 20% of stroke patients and may be indicative of a behavioural or emotional expression of an underlying depression associated with anterior cortical or subcortical damage.

SSRIs, the half-lives of sertraline and citalopram are prolonged in the elderly. If a tricyclic antidepressant is required, nortriptyline may be better tolerated. Amoxapine should be avoided because of its potential for causing EPS in this at risk population, as should tricyclics with a greater degree of anticholinergic activity. Trazodone and nefazodone may also be antidepressants of choice because they have fewer cardiac and anticholinergic effects. Orthostatic hypotension may need to be monitored, however. MAOIs should be avoided because of their propensity to cause orthostatic hypotension and because the dietary restrictions may be difficult to follow for some.

❖ *Electroconvulsive therapy (ECT)* is a safe and effective treatment option in this population for severe depression and for mania and may be better tolerated than pharmacotherapy in some patients.

❖ For late-onset *bipolar disorder*, lithium appears to be as effective as in early-onset cases, but long-term follow-up studies have not been done to date. Lithium toxicity may occur at levels that would be considered 'therapeutic' in younger patients. Lithium clearance is reduced in the elderly and doses may be upto 50% lower. Of AED mood stabilisers, carbamazepine has more adverse cardiac effects and needs to be monitored with ECGs in the elderly and sodium valproate may thus be preferred. The half-life of valproate may be longer in the elderly and the free fraction may also be increased.

❖ The elderly are much more susceptible to the extrapyramidal symptoms (EPS) of *antipsychotics* as well as to the orthostatic hypotension and anticholinergic effects of these agents. When indicated they should be used in much lower doses (generally one half to one third of doses in younger adults) and titrated more slowly with frequent monitoring. It is useful to monitor the elderly for Parkinsonian side effects and for tardive dyskinesia on a three monthly basis and more frequently at the onset of therapy or when making dose adjustments. Clozapine may be associated with an increased incidence of agranulocytosis in the elderly and anecdotally has not been thought as effective as in younger adults. Sertindole should not be used in the elderly because of its cardiac effects and drug interactions. Risperidone may be used in the elderly, but its half life may be increased and blood pressure should be monitored. The lesser cardiac, anticholinergic and extrapyramidal effects of sulpiride and olanzapine make these drugs of choice in this population.

❖ *Benzodiazepines* and *drugs with a high degree of anticholinergic activity* should be avoided.

Use of Psychotropics Following Stroke

Psychotropic classification	Recommended drugs
Antidepressants	Moclobemide SSRIs
Antipsychotics	Olanzapine Risperidone Sulpiride
Mood stabilisers	Lithium Sodium Valproate

VI

Management of
Medical/Psychiatric
Emergencies

Management of Simple Paracetamol Poisoning

This protocol is suitable for poisoning with paracetamol alone. Do not use this protocol if you suspect another substance has been taken in excess

---

1
* Do not induce vomiting
* Do not give activated charcoal
(both actions may lessen the effect of any methionine given)

2
* If amount of paracetamol taken is more than 150mg/kg or is not known: <u>give methionine 10 tablets, stat.</u> and arrange for immediate transfer to district general hospital. **Do not** follow this protocol.

* If amount taken is known to be less than 150mg/kg, follow protocol below

---

3
* If amount taken is known to be *less than* 150mg/kg -
<u>give methionine 10 x 250mg tablets immediately</u>
DO NOT DELAY

4
* Take blood sample <u>*four hours*</u> after overdose or as soon after this as possible.
(If plasma level determination cannot be done urgently (to allow treatment within 8 hours of ingestion) - transfer to DGH)
* Check result against graph in the BNF (Section - 'Emergency Treatment of Poisoning')

5
i) If levels below 'normal' treatment line **and** patient not anorexic (BMI <17.5), HIV +ve, alcoholic or on enzyme inducers:
No further treatment required.
ii) If levels above normal treatment line **and** asymptomatic (no nausea/vomiting) **and** less than ten hours since ingestion:
continue with oral methionine - give three further doses of 2.5g (every four hours). Check INR/LFTs.
iii) If patient fails any criteria in (i) or (ii), or if in **any doubt** discuss with medical team at DGH with a view to urgent transfer.
iv) If ingestion is > 24 hrs ago, consult poisons information service immediately.

Rapid Tranquillisation

Algorithm for rapid control of the acutely disturbed patient

(This algorithm is for guidance only: rigid adherence to it may not always be appropriate)

Consider non-drug measures: talking-down, distraction, seclusion. Try *oral* therapy

↓ No response

Give either:
Haloperidol 5-10mg IV + diazepam 10mg IV
Wait ten minutes
OR
Droperidol 5-10mg IM + lorazepam 2mg IM
Wait thirty minutes

→ Response → Consider starting/increasing regular *oral* medication

↓ No response

Repeat above
Wait ten minutes for IV
OR
Thirty minutes for IM
May repeat again
up to a maximum of 60mg haloperidol + 60 mg diazepam,

→ Response → (Re)commence oral antipsychotics
OR
Give zuclopenthixol acetate (Clopixol Acuphase) 50-150mg.
Peaks at 24-36 hours; effective for 72 hours

↓ No response

→ Response → As above

Notes:

* Seek advice from your consultant at any stage if you are in any doubt

* Monitor respiratory rate, pulse, BP, every 5 mins
* Benzodiazepines safer than antipsychotics but beware of accumulation. Use benzos alone if any cardiac disease.
* Never give Clopixol Acuphase to a struggling patient or to those who are antipsychotic naive.
* Procyclidine IV/IM must be available – ? give as prophylaxis

* Facilities for mechanical ventilation/cardiac resus must be available
* If contact with patient is lost: monitor as for full anaesthetic procedure – use Pulse Oximeter
* Give flumazenil if respiratory rate drops below 10/minute
* Use IV route if IM is ineffective after three doses

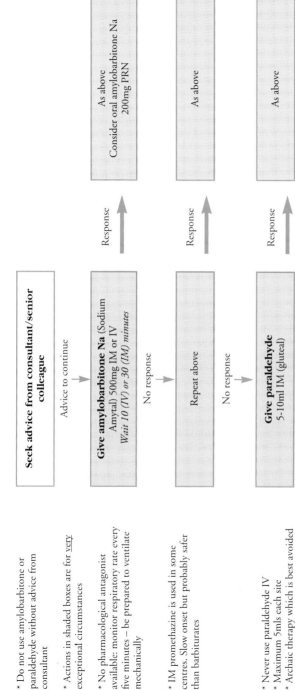

* Do not use amylobarbitone or paraldehyde without advice from consultant

* Actions in shaded boxes are for <u>very</u> exceptional circumstances

* No pharmacological antagonist available: monitor respiratory rate every five minutes – be prepared to ventilate mechanically

* IM promethazine is used in some centres. Slow onset but probably safer than barbiturates

* Never use paraldehyde IV
* Maximum 5mls each site
* Archaic therapy which is best avoided

Seek advice from consultant/senior colleague

Advice to continue

Give amylobarbitone Na (Sodium Amytal) 500mg IM or IV
Wait 10 (IV) or 30 (IM) minutes

No response

Repeat above

No response

Give paraldehyde 5-10ml IM (gluteal)

Response → As above. Consider oral amylobarbitone Na 200mg PRN

Response → As above

Response → As above

Maximum rates of **IV** administration: amylobarbitone 50mg/min; diazepam 5mg/min; droperidol, haloperidol, lorazepam – give over 2-3 minutes.
<u>Never mix lorazepam or diazepam with other drugs in the same syringe</u>
<u>Never give diazepam IM</u>

Adapted from: Kerr I, Taylor D (1997). Acute disturbed or violent behaviour: principals of treatment. Journal of Psychopharmacology, 11, 271-277.

VII

Adverse Effects of

Psychotropic Drugs

Guidelines for the Management of Weight Change in Patients on Psychotropic Medication

General Considerations:

✦ Weight change is a common problem in patients on psychotropic medication with weight gain occurring in approximately 60% of patients on lithium, and 25-50% of patients on valproate, antipsychotics and antidepressants.

✦ Weight gain generally occurs because calorie intake exceeds calorie expenditure. This may occur because of actions on a variety of receptors, which can affect hunger and thirst mechanisms, carbohydrate and lipid storage and other metabolic factors. Adverse effects of the drugs may also play a role eg. lithium-induced hypothyroidism, sedation caused by some antipsychotics. In most instances of weight change with psychotropics, the mechanism remains to be elucidated.

✦ Weight gain and weight loss have potentially serious health ramifications in addition to the cosmetic distress often expressed by the patient and is also a frequent cause of poor compliance of medications. The patient's concerns about weight change with respect to their medication should be asked about routinely in all patients on psychotropic medication. Patients are often unwell at the start of treatment, so this discussion should continue as they recover. Motivation and degree of concern about weight are key factors in determining compliance and should be discussed.

✦ When considering a subjective complaint of weight change, it is important to consider the natural history of the illness itself, the temporal relationship of the weight problem as well as the relative weight change with respect to height and to original and ideal or 'healthy' body weight.

✦ It is important to consider other possible causes in the management of suspected weight change in patients on psychotropics. TSH should be measured, as thyroid abnormalities may be associated with various mental state changes and as some drugs may cause thyroid dysfunction (e.g. carbamazepine, lithium). Some other aetiologies for weight change which should be considered include the following:

weight loss: anorexia nervosa, hypophagia due to depression, delusions concerning food in psychosis, obsessions or ruminations about food in anxiety disorders, underlying neoplasia or other serious medical illness, thyroid dysfunction, unusually restrictive diets

weight gain: hyperphagia occurring in depression or related to psychosocial stresses, weight gain occurring as a normal part of recovery in depression, thyroid dysfunction, recent smoking discontinuation, oedema or ascites from medical illness (primary or secondary to effects of medications), polydipsia (related to medical or psychiatric illness or to the effects of medication), pregnancy (occurring independently of medication or secondary to oral contraceptive failure due to enzyme-inducing agents e.g. carbamazepine)

✦ Consider risk factors, where known. Lithium and valproate have weight gain associated with a predisposition to gain weight, female sex and dose and duration of therapy. Risk factors for antidepressants and antipsychotics have not been yet elucidated.

✦ Consider the individual risk of a given drug for weight change (see table).

✦ All weight changes thought secondary to psychotropics should be discussed fully with the patient. Discussion should continue through recovery, as they may be unwell at the start of therapy. Weight gain from psychotropics often plateaus after a few months and it may thus not always be helpful to switch to an alternative psychotropic. If it is decided to switch to an alternative treatment because of weight change, the patient must be informed of the risk of illness relapse and of other side effects with alternative medications before hand.

✦ Stimulants and other anorexants are not recommended as treatment for side effects of weight gain with psychotropics. Surgical strategies are also not generally recommended as a solution. The use of fluoxetine or of orlistat (tetrahydrolipstatin) may be possible interventions, but neither has been evaluated in this clinical situation.

✦ The use of steroids or body building preparations are not recommended in the treatment of weight loss as a side effect of psychotropics. Such preparations may exacerbate psychiatric symptoms in addition to their other well-known side effects. Patients should be referred wherever possible to a dietician for management of weight loss.

✦ Patients should be referred to a dietician for weight change related to psychotropics, mental status allowing. The patient must also be motivated for such a referral. Fad diets should be avoided. Low fat, high fibre diets maximising fruits and vegetables and complex (over simple) carbohydrates are recommended. Frequency of eating should be considered and thirst as a side effect should be identified, addressing consumption of sugary drinks specifically. This may be a particular risk factor for weight gain with lithium, but may also occur with other medications. As concordance with diets is often difficult, this is best done in conjunction with a behavioural programme and with biofeedback where appropriate.

✦ Exercise is also essential for the management of weight gain: 10-15 minutes/ day of exercise may assist the weight loss regime and is best worked into the patient's usual activities of daily living.

Psychotropics and Weight Change

Drug Class	Drugs causing weight gain	Drugs causing weight loss	Drugs thought not to influence weight
Antidepressants	Amitriptyline Imipramine, other TCAs Isocarboxazid Phenelzine ?Tranylcypromine	Fluoxetine ? Bupropion	SSRIs, Moclobemide Venlafaxine Trazodone Nefazodone Amoxapine
Antipsychotics	Phenothiazines Depot preparations Haloperidol Clozapine Olanzapine Quetiapine Risperidone	None	Molindone (not available in UK) Loxapine ?Perphenazine Ziprasidone (not available yet)
Anxiolytics	None	None	Benzodiazepines
Mood Stabilisers / Antiepileptic Drugs	Lithium Sodium Valproate Vigabatrin ?Carbamazepine	Topiramate, Felbamate	Lamotrigine Gabapentin Phenobarbitone Phenytoin
Stimulants	None	Amphetamines Methylphenidate	? Modafinil

✦ *Antidepressants:* The previous reports of body weight increase by antidepressants were probably overestimates of the problem as weight gain may be a normal part of recovery from depression in some individuals. While one third to one half of patients on tricyclics may experience weight gain, this is usually only modest. Amitriptyline appears to carry the highest risk of TCAs. The non-selective MAOIs also carry significant risk of weight gain and these effects may be additive if used in conjunction with a tricyclic. If weight gain persists, an SSRI or reversible inhibitor of MAO-A (moclobemide) should be considered. Care must be taken to follow the guidelines for switching between these agents. Weight loss appearing during the course of depression is more likely to be related to hypophagia associated with the illness than to be drug-related.

✦ *Mood stabilisers / Antiepileptic Drugs:* Weight gain associated with valproate and lithium as mood stabilisers is common and frequently affects patient concordance with these agents. Although serum lithium levels over 0.8 mmol/L are associated with weight gain, lowering of lithium below these levels as a means of weight management cannot be recommended routinely as they will be clinically suboptimal in most patients. Those with identified risk factors should be considered as candidates for carbamazepine, which is less likely to induce weight gain. Thyroid function tests should be checked on any patient on lithium or carbamazepine experiencing weight gain. Lamotrigine and gabapentin are not associated with significant weight gain, but there are too few data concerning their efficacy as mood stabilisers to recommend switching to these agents routinely. The data concerning other AEDs as mood stabilisers are even less convincing.

✦   *Antipsychotics:* Phenothiazines and the newer atypical agents appear to have the greatest risk of weight gain associated with their use. Some have suggested that there is a correlation between treatment efficacy and bodyweight gain for many antipsychotics. There is a theoretical problem with the common use of valproate with clozapine as both may cause significant weight gain, although no clinical studies have addressed this potential problem to date. Of the typical antipsychotics, butyrophenones are less likely than phenothiazines to cause body weight gain and loxapine, molindone and perphenazine do not appear to cause weight gain, although data are scarce.

✦   *Anxiolytics:* Consistent weight changes with anxiolytics have not been demonstrated, and other causes should be sought when weight change occurs in this clinical situation (eg. co-morbidty with an eating disorder or depression; eg. thyroid disorder causing anxiety symptoms).

✦   *Stimulants:* Amphetamines and methylphenidate frequently cause weight loss; modafinil has been reported to cause anorexia more commonly than placebo, but there are few data relevant to weight changes with this agent.

Specific recommendations:

On initial prescription of psychotropics likely to cause weight change:

(1) consider risk factors,

(2) discuss pros and cons with patient,

(3) monitor weight monthly x 6 months then every 3 months,

(4) consider early referral to a dietician, if patient agreeable and mental state appropriate

(5) consider the possible additive effects of weight change effects if this psychotropic is being added to another producing similar weight change

(6) obtain baseline BMI and relevant laboratory parameters (eg. TFTs)

(7) consider the patient's ideal body weight, any other risk factors for obesity-related illness and the attitude of the patient towards weight gain or loss

---

If weight change does occur, rule out other possible causes:

(1)   take careful history, including dietary and family history as well as temporal relationship of weight change to initiation and dose changes of psychotropics

(2)   consider the role of thirst which should not be underestimated – in particular all drinks with high sugar content should be excluded

(3)   physical examination to include height, weight, calculation of body mass index; look for evidence of ascites, myxoedema

(4)   check thyroid function tests, FBC, LFTs, albumin, electrolytes

(5)   consider other relevant tests, eg. pregnancy testing

156

If other causes of weight change excluded, institute dietary and exercise regime in conjunction with dietician and/or exercise physiologist. Ideally, such exercise should be undertaken in groups as the psychological benefits of such encouragement are important. The types of exercise chosen must take into account any effects of the medication on alertness or coordination.

If above not successful, consider alternative drugs in same class which might have less risk for weight change (see table). However, weight gain often plateaus and so switching may not always be necessary or desirable. Any such change that does occur must take into account the risk of relapse on changing of medication and be fully discussed with the patient with respect to risks and benefits.

Antidepressants – Relative Adverse Effects

Drug	Sedation	Cardio-Toxicity	Anti-Cholinergic Effects	Forms available
Tricyclics				
Imipramine	++	+++	+++	tabs, liq
Amitriptyline	+++	+++	+++	tabs/caps, liq, inj
Desipramine*	+	++	+	tabs
Nortriptyline	+	++	+	tabs
Trimipramine	+++	+++	++	tabs, caps
Doxepin	+++	++	++	caps
Dothiepin	+++	+++	++	tabs, caps
Clomipramine	++	+++	++	tabs/caps, liq, inj
Lofepramine	+	+	+	tabs
Atypical Antidepressants				
Mirtazapine	+++	- ?	+	tabs
Nefazodone	++	-	-	tabs
Reboxetine	+	- ?	+	tabs
Trazodone	+++	+	-	caps, liq
Venlafaxine	++	- ?	+	tabs
Selective Serotonin Reuptake Inhibitors (SSRIs)				
Citalopram	-	- ?	-	tabs
Fluvoxamine	+	- ?	-	tabs
Fluoxetine	-	-	-	caps, liq
Sertraline	-	-	-	tabs
Paroxetine	+	-	+	tabs, liq
Monoamine Oxidase Inhibitors (MAOIs)				
Isocarboxazid	+	++	++	tabs
Phenelzine	+	+	+	tabs
Tranylcypromine	-	+	+	tabs
Reversible Inhibitor Of Monoamine Oxidase A (RIMA)				
Moclobemide	-	-	-	tabs

KEY: +++ High incidence/severity   - Very low/none
       ++ Moderate   + Low
* In UK, available on named – patient basis only

Antipsychotics-Adverse Effects

Antipsychotics-Relative Adverse Effects

Drug	Sedation	Extra-pyramidal	Anti-muscarinic	Hypotension	Cardiac toxicity	Prolactin elevation
Chlorpromazine	+++	++	++	+++	++	+++
Promazine	+++	+	++	++	+	++
Thioridazine	+++	+	+++	+++	+++	++
Fluphenazine	+	+++	++	+	+	+++
Perphenazine	+	+++	+	+	+	+++
Trifluoperazine	+	+++	+/ -	+	+	+++
Flupenthixol	+	++	++	+	+	+++
Zuclopenthixol	++	++	++	+	+	+++
Haloperidol	+	+++	+	+	+	+++
Droperidol	++	+++	+	+	+	+++
Benperidol	+	+++	+	+	+	+++
Sulpiride	-	+	+/ -	-	-	+++
Pimozide	+	+	+	+	+++	+++
Loxapine	++	+++	+	++	+	+++
Clozapine	+++	-	+++	+++	+	-
Risperidone	+	+	+	++	-	+++
Sertindole*	-	-	-	+++	+++	-
Olanzapine	++	+/ -	+	+	-	+
Quetiapine	++	-	+	++	-	-
Amisulpride	-	+	-	-	-	+++

Key: +++ High incidence/ severity ++ Moderate
+ Low - Very low
* Named patient only

Clozapine: Management Of Adverse Effects

Adverse effect	Timecourse	Action
Sedation	First 4 weeks. May persist, but usually wears off.	Give smaller dose in the mornings. Some patients can only cope with single night-time dosing. Reduce dose if necessary.
Hypersalivation	First 4 weeks. May persist, but usually wears off. Often very troublesome at night.	Give hyoscine 300mcg (Kwells) sucked and swallowed at night. Pirenzepine (not licensed in the UK) up to 50mg tds may be tried. Patients do not always mind excess salivation: treatment not always required.
Constipation	Usually persists	Recommend high fibre diet. Bulk forming laxatives +/-stimulants may be used.
Hypotension	First 4 weeks	Advise patient to take time when standing up. Reduce dose or slow down rate of increase. If severe, consider moclobemide and Bovril, or fludrocortisone.
Hypertension	First 4 weeks, sometimes longer	Monitor closely and increase dose as slowly as is necessary. Hypotensive therapy (e.g. atenolol 25mg/day) is rarely necessary.
Tachycardia	First 4 weeks, but often persists.	Often occurs if dose escalation is too rapid. Inform patient that it is not dangerous. Give small dose of beta-blocker if necessary.
Weight gain	Usually during the first year of treatment	Dietary counselling is essential. Advice may be more effective if given before weight gain occurs. Weight gain is common and often profound (10lbs +)
Fever	First 3 weeks	Give antipyretic but check FBC. NB. This fever is not usually related to blood dyscrasias.
Seizures	May occur at any time	Dose /dose increase related. Consider prophylactic valproate* if on high dose. After a seizure – withhold clozapine for one day. Restart at reduced dose. Give sodium valproate.
Nausea	First 6 weeks	May give anti-emetic. Avoid prochlorperazine and metoclopramide (EPSE).
Nocturnal enuresis	May occur at any time	Try manipulating dose schedule. Avoid fluids before bedtime. In severe cases, desmopressin is usually effective.
Neutropenia/ agranulocytosis	First 18 weeks (but may occur at any time)	Stop clozapine; admit to hospital.

* Usual dose is 1000-2000mg/day. Plasma levels may be useful as a rough guide to dosing – aim for 50-100mg/l. Use of modified release preparation (Epilim Chrono) may aid compliance: can be given once daily and may be better tolerated.

Algorithm for the Treatment of Antipsychotic-Induced Akathisia

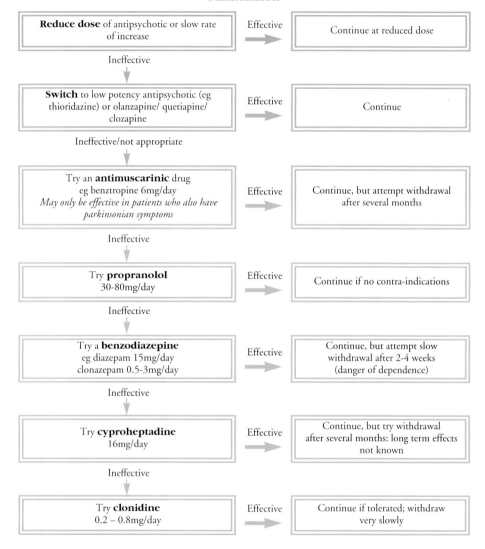

Reduce dose of antipsychotic or slow rate of increase	Effective →	Continue at reduced dose

Ineffective ↓

Switch to low potency antipsychotic (eg thioridazine) or olanzapine/ quetiapine/ clozapine	Effective →	Continue

Ineffective/not appropriate ↓

Try an **antimuscarinic** drug eg benztropine 6mg/day *May only be effective in patients who also have parkinsonian symptoms*	Effective →	Continue, but attempt withdrawal after several months

Ineffective ↓

Try **propranolol** 30-80mg/day	Effective →	Continue if no contra-indications

Ineffective ↓

Try a **benzodiazepine** eg diazepam 15mg/day clonazepam 0.5-3mg/day	Effective →	Continue, but attempt slow withdrawal after 2-4 weeks (danger of dependence)

Ineffective ↓

Try **cyproheptadine** 16mg/day	Effective →	Continue, but try withdrawal after several months: long term effects not known

Ineffective ↓

Try **clonidine** 0.2 – 0.8mg/day	Effective →	Continue if tolerated; withdraw very slowly

Notes:

*Akathisia is sometimes difficult to diagnose with certainty. A careful history of symptoms and drug use is essential. Note that severe akathisia may be linked to violent behaviour.
*Evaluate efficacy of each treatment option over at least one month. Some effect may be seen after a few days but it may take much longer to become apparent in those with chronic akathisia.
* Withdraw previously ineffective treatments before starting the next option in the algorithm.
* Consider tardive akathisia in patients on long term therapy.

Algorithm for the Treatment of Symptomatic, Antipsychotic-Induced Hyperprolactinaemia

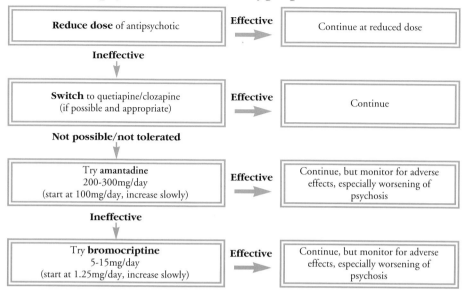

Notes:

* Hyperprolactinaemia is often asymptomatic. Adverse effects, when they do occur, are usually mild and do not affect quality of life. Remedial treatment is therefore only rarely appropriate. In cases of apparent infertility, specialist advice should be sought.
* Before starting treatment – take a full sexual/menstrual history to establish whether or not symptoms are related to antipsychotic use.
* Other causes of hyperprolactinaemia (eg prolactin-secreting tumour) must be considered.
* Evaluate efficacy of each treatment option over at least one month: prolactin levels may fall within days but adverse effects such as gynaecomastia respond more slowly.
* Withdraw previously ineffective treatments before starting the next option in the algorithm.
* Olanzapine causes dose-dependent, transient hyperprolactinaemia. Symptoms are rare, especially at 10mg/day.

Modified from Duncan and Taylor (1995)

The Neuroleptic Malignant Syndrome

*   Incidence: 0.5 – 1% patients

*   Mortality (untreated) 20%

*   Onset may be acute or insidious

*   Course may fluctuate

*   May occur out of hospital

SIGNS AND SYMPTOMS

- intense diaphoresis
- fever/hyperthermia
- hypertension/autonomic instability (fluctuating B.P.)
- tachycardia
- incontinence / retention / obstruction
- muscular rigidity (may be confined to head and neck)
- confusion, agitation/altered consciousness
- raised creatinine phosphokinase > 1000 IU/L (controversial)
- leukocytosis

RISK FACTORS

- organic brain disease: alcoholism, dementia
- hypermetabolic states: hyperthyroidism
- psychiatric diagnosis
- Parkinsons' disease
- agitation
- dehydration
- history of catatonia
- high dose antipsychotic
- recent dose increase

PRECIPITATING FACTORS

- antipsychotics: typical and atypical
- rapidity of titration and dose of drug
- antipsychotic withdrawal
- antidepressants: including SSRIs
- abrupt cessation of dopamine agonists
- other drugs: tetrabenazine
- drugs of abuse: cocaine, MDMA, amphetamine

163

TREATMENTS

✦ withdraw antipsychotic immediately
✦ general supportive medical intervention on medical ward
✦ rehydration
✦ sedation with short-acting benzodiazepines
✦ dopamine agonists: bromocriptine, dantrolene
✦ antimuscarinic agents
✦ propranolol
✦ electroconvulsive therapy
✦ plasmaphoresis

COMPLICATIONS

✦ renal: rhabdomyolysis leading to renal failure
✦ cardiovascular: arrythmias, cardiac arrest, stroke, cardiogenic shock
✦ respiratory: respiratory failure, pulmonary embolus
✦ hepatic failure
✦ E.coli fasciitis

Antipsychotic Rechallenge

❑ antipsychotic rechallenge following NMS is associated with an acceptable risk in most patients

❑ gender and age do not affect successful rechallenge

❑ a minimum of 5-14 days should elapse post recovery

❑ generally, successful rechallenge uses structurally dissimilar agents

❑ lower doses are recommended, with extremely slow titration

❑ depot preparations should be avoided

❑ agents with lower D_2 receptor blockade may be preferred, but data are inconclusive

Algorithm for the Treatment of Tardive Dyskinesia (TD)

Prevention whenever possible	* consider risk factors e.g. females, the elderly, affective disorder, total antipsychotic dose - use lowest dose of antipsychotic for shortest time necessary - reasses need for antipsychotic regularly e.g. three monthly - reasses need for antimuscarinic regularly - consider use of antipsychotic less likely to cause TD
If TD develops withdraw any antimuscarinic Consider withdrawing antipsychotic slowly	* antimuscarinic withdrawal may allow improvement in TD * balance risk of relapse against risk of TD * TD is not usually progressive * continuing at the lowest possible dose minimises the risk of progression

Antipsychotic required

If antipsychotic necessary consider clozapine or olanzapine	* clozapine may allow improvement in TD * consider using mood stabilisers alone for bipolar disorder * theoretical reasons for using risperidone or quetiapine

Further measures

Consider Vitamin E 400 iu/day; may increase by 400iu weekly to a maximum of 1600iu/day in divided doses	* consider withdrawing other drugs which may cause or exacerbate movement disorders e.g. metoclopramide, antidepressants, stimulants, antimuscarinics and antiparkinsonian agents

TD persists

* monitor for GI effects of Vitamin E
* treatment duration is not clearly established

Consider clonazepam 1mg/day (elderly 0.5mg) and ↑ over 2-4 weeks to 4.5mg/day	* tolerance to clonazepam may develop; therefore intermittent treatment is preferable *dystonia may respond better

TD persists

* Other proposed treatments Consider: * Nifedipine 40 – 80mg[1]/day * Sodium Valproate[2] * Propanolol – for tardive akathisia * Botulinum toxin – for tardive dystonia * Tetrabenazine – A/E limit use e.g. depression * Increasing antipsychotic dose[3]	1. maybe more effective in elderly and in severe TD 2. some evidence of efficacy ?prophylactic use 3. will improve TD initially but will worsen TD in long term

N.B. Symptoms of TD occur in untreated schizophrenia: antipsychotics are not the only risk factor.
** Modified from Duncan et al., 1997.

Key References

Key References

Key References

Space does not permit the listing of all references used in developing the treatment guidelines set out in this book. We have, however, listed below some of the more influential papers used. This list gives a fair representation of the literature background to the Prescribing Guidelines and affords readers a starting point in their own investigations.

Principles of Psychotropic Prescribing

American Psychiatric Association (1996) Practice Guidelines, APPress, Washington, DC., USA

Aravagiri, M., Ames, D., Wirshing, W.C., et al (1996) Plasma level monitoring of olanzapine in patients with schizophrenia: determination by high-performance liquid chromatography with electrochemical detection. *Therapeutic Drug Monitoring*, **19**, 307-313.

British Medical Association, Royal Pharmaceutical Society of Great Britain (1998) British National Formulary 36, *BMA / RPSGB*, London, U.K.

Ginestet, D. (1996) Guide du Bon Usage des Psychotropes, Doin Editeurs, Paris, France

Kaplan, H.I., Sadock, B.J. (1996) Pocket Handbook of Psychiatric Drug Treatment, American Psychiatric Press, Washington DC., U.S.A.

Kilpatrick, E.S., Forrest, G., Brodie, M.J. (1996) Concentration-effect and concentration-toxicity relations with lamotrigine: a prospective study. *Epilepsia*, **37**, 534-538.

McConnell, H. (1998) Psychological and Behavioral Correlates of Blood and CSF Laboratory Tests. In: PJ Snyder & PD Nussbaum (Eds), Clinical Neuropsychology for House Staff, American Psychological Press, Washington, U.S.A.

McConnell, H., Bianchine, J. (1994) Cerebrospinal Fluid in Neurology and Psychiatry. Chapman Hall, London, U.K.

McConnell, H., Andrews, C. (1999) The EEG in Psychiatry. In: *Clinical Neurophysiology*. C. Binnie (ed), Blackwell, Oxford, U.K.

McConnell, H., Snyder, P.J. (1998) Electroencephalography in the elderly. In: P.Nussbaum (Ed.), Handbook of Neuropsychology and Aging. A volume in the *Critical Issues in Neuropsychology* series (E.E. Puente & C.R. Reynolds, Eds.). New York: Plenum Press.

Perry, P.J., Miller, D.D., Arndt, S.V., et al (1991) Clozapine and norclozapine plasma concentrations and clinical response of treatment refractory schizophrenic patients. *American Journal of Psychiatry*, **148**, 231-235.

Potkin, S.G., Bera, R., Gulasekaram, B., et al (1994) Plasma clozapine concentrations predict clinical response in treatment-resitant schizophrenia. *Journal of Clinical Psychiatry*, **55** (Suppl. 9B), 133-136.

Rosse, R.B., Giese, A., Deutsch, S., Morihisa, J.M. (1989) Laboratory Diagnostic Testing in Psychiatry, American Psychiatric Press, Washington DC, U.S.A.

Smith, P., Darlington, C. (1996) Clinical Psychopharmacology. Lawrence Erlbaum Associates, Mahwah, NJ, U.S.A.

Snyder, P.J. & McConnell, H. (1998) Epilepsy in the Elderly. In: P. Nussbaum (Ed.) Handbook of Neuropsychology and Aging. A volume in the *Critical Issues in Neuropsychology* series (A.E. Puente & C.R. Reynolds, Eds.). Plenum Press, New York, U.S.A.

Taylor, D.M., Duncan, D. (1995). The use of clozapine plasma levels in optimising therapy. *Psychiatric Bulletin*, **19**, 753-755.

Taylor, D., Duncan, D. (1997) Doses of carbamazepine and valproate in bipolar affective disorder. *Psychiatric Bulletin*, **21**, 221-223.

Taylor, D., Paton C. (1998) Case studies in Psychopharmacolgy: The Use of Drugs in Psychiatry, Martin Dunitz, London, U.K.

Victorian Drug Usage Advisory Committee (1995) Psychotropic Drug Guidelines, VMPF Therapeutics Committee, Victoria, Australia.

Treatment of Psychosis and Schizophrenia

Boyer, P., Lecrubier, Y., Puech, A.J. *et al*. (1995) Treatment of negative symptoms in schizophrenia with amisulpride. *British Journal of Psychiatry*, **166**, 68-72.

Conley, R.R., Tamminga, C.A., Bartko, J.J. *et al.* (1998) Olanzapine compared with chlorpromazine in treatment-resistant schizophrenia. *American Journal of Psychiatry*, **155**, 914-920.

Duncan, D., McConnell, H., Taylor, D. (1997) Tardive dyskinesia: how is it prevented and treated? *Psychiatric Bulletin*, **21**, 422-425.

Henderson, D.C., Nasrallah, R.A., Goff, D.C. (1998) Switching from clozapine to olanzapine in treatment-refractory schizophrenia: safety, clinical efficacy, and predictors of response. *Journal of Clinical Psychiatry*, **59**, 585-588.

Kane, J.M., Honingfeld, G., Singer, J. *et al.* (1988). Clozapine for the treatment-resistant schizophrenic: a double blind comparison. *Archives of General Psychiatry*, **45**, 789-796.

Mir, S., Taylor, D. (1998) Schizophrenia. *The Pharmaceutical Journal*, **261**, 55-58.

Morris, S., Hogan, T., McGuire, A. (1998) The cost-effectiveness of clozapine: a survey of the literature. *Clinical Drug Investigations*, **15**, 137-152.

O'Brien, J., Barber, R. (1998) Marked improvement in tardive dyskinesia following treatment with olanzapine in an elderly subject. *British Journal of Psychiatry*, **172**, 186-189.

Rosenheck, R., Cramer, J., Xu, W. *et al.* (1997) A comparison of clozapine and haloperidol in hospitalized patients with refractory schizophrenia. *The New England Journal of Medicine*, **337**, 809-815.

Sheitman, B.B., Lindgren, J.C., Early, J. (1997) High-dose olanzapine for treatment-refractory schizophrenia. *American Journal of Psychiatry*, **154**, 1626.

Siris, S.G. (1993). Adjunctive medication in the maintenance treatment of schizophrenia and its conceptual implications. *British Journal of Psychiatry*, **163** [Suppl 22], 66-78.

Taylor, D.M., Duncan, D. (1995). The use of clozapine plasma levels in optimising therapy. *Psychiatric Bulletin*, **19**, 753-755.

Taylor D. (1997) Monitoring the new atypical antipsychotic drugs. *Progress in Neurology and Psychiatry*, **1(3)**, 13-15.

Thompson, C. (1994). The use of high-dose antipsychotic medication. *British Journal of Psychiatry*, **164**, 448-458.

Tollefson, G.D., Beasley Jr, C.M., Tran, P.V. *et al.* (1997) Olanzapine versus haloperidol in the treatment of schizophrenia and schizoaffective and schizophreniform disorders: results of an international collaborative trial. *American Journal of Psychiatry*, **154**, 457-465.

Equivalent doses of antipsychotics

Bazire, S. (1999) *Psychotropic Drug Directory*. Quay Books Division, Dinton, Wilts, U.K.

Foster, P. (1989) Neuroleptic equivalence. *Pharmaceutical Journal*, **290**, 431-432

Treatment of Affective Disorder

Depression

Austin, M.P.V., Sonza, F.G.N., Goodwin, G.M. (1991). Lithium augmentation in antidepressant resistant patients. A quantitative analysis. *British Journal of Psychiatry*, **159**, 510-514.

Brown, T.M., Skop, B.P., Mareth, T.R. (1996) Pathophysiology and management of the serotonin syndrome. *Annals of Pharmacotherapy*, **30**, 527-533.

Checkley, S. (ed) (1998) *The Management of Depression*. Blackwell Science Ltd., Oxford, U.K.

Dimitriou, E.C., Dimitriou, C.E. (1998) Buspirone augmentation of antidepressant therapy. *Journal of Clinical Psychopharmacology*, **18**, 465-469.

Dinan, T.G., Lavelle, E., Cooney, J. *et al.* (1997). Dexamethasone augmentation in treatment-resistant depression. *Acta Psychiatrica Scandinavica*, **95**, 58-61.

Goodwin, F.K., Prange, A.J., Post, R.M., *et al.* (1982). Potentiation of antidepressant effects of L-triiodothyronine in tricyclic nonresponders. *American Journal of Psychiatry*, **139**, 34-38.

Haddad, P. (1997) Newer antidepressants and the discontinuation syndrome. *Journal of Clinical Psychiatry*, **58** (Suppl. 7), 17-22.

Lane, R., Baldwin, D. (1997) Selective serotonin reuptake inhibitor-induced serotonin syndrome: review. *Journal of Clinical Psychopharmacology*, **17**, 208-221.

McAskill, R., Mir, S., Taylor, D. (1998) Pindolol augmentation of antidepressant therapy. *British Journal of Psychiatry*, **173**, 203-208.

Sternbach, H. (1991) The serotonin syndrome. *American Journal of Psychiatry*, **148**, 705-713.

Taylor, D. (1995). Selective serotonin reuptake inhibitors and tricyclic antidepressants in combination. Interactions and therapeutic uses. *British Journal of Psychiatry*, **167**, 575-580.

Zajecka, J., Tracy, K.A., Mitchell, S. (1997) Discontinuation symptoms after treatment with serotonin reuptake inhibitors: a literature review. *Journal of Clinical Psychiatry*, **58**, 291-297.

Zanardi, R., Franchini, L., Gasperini,M., *et al* (1998) Faster onset of action of fluvoxamine in combination with pindolol in the treatment of delusional depression: a controlled study. *Journal of Clinical Psychopharmacology*, **18**, 441-446.

ECT

Bazire, S. (1999) *Psychotropic Drug Directory*. Quay Books Division, Dinton, Wilts, U.K.

Curran, S., Freeman, C.P. (1995) ECT and drugs. In: Freeman, C.P.(ed). *The ECT Handbook – The second report of the Royal College of Psychiatrists' special committee on ECT*. Henry Ling Ltd., Dorset Press, U.K.

Jarvis, M.R., Goewert, A.J., Zorumski, C.F. (1992). Novel antidepressants and maintenance electroconvulsive therapy. *Annals of Clinical Psychiatry*, **4**, 275-284.

Kellner, C.H., Nixon, D.W., Bernstein, H.J. (1991) ECT- Drug interactions: a review. *Psychopharmacology Bulletin*, **27**, 595-609.

Maidment, I. (1997) The interaction between psychiatric medicines and ECT. *Hospital Pharmacist,* **4**, 102-105.

Welch, C.A. (1995) Electroconvulsive therapy. In: Ciraulo, D.A., Shader, R.I., Greenblatt, D.J., Creelman, W. (ed). *Drug Interactions in Psychiatry – 2nd edition*. Williams & Wilkins.

Bipolar affective disorder

Calabrese, J.R., Meltzer, H.Y., Markovitz, P.J. (1991). Clozapine prophylaxis in rapid cycling bipolar disorder. *Journal of Clinical Psychopharmacology*, **11**, 396-397.

Calabrese, J.R., Woyshville, M.J. (1995). A medication algorithm for treatment of bipolar rapid cycling? *Journal of Clinical Psychiatry*, **56** [suppl 3], 11-18.

Duncan, D., McConnell, H.W., Taylor, D. (1998) Lamotrigine in bipolar affective disorder. *Psychiatric Bulletin*, **22**, 630-632.

Goodnick, P.J. (1995). Nimodipine treatment of rapid cycling bipolar disorder. *Journal of Clinical Psychiatry*, **56**, 330.

McConnell, H.W., Duncan, D. (1998a) *Behavioural effects of antiepileptic drugs*. In: Psychiatric co-morbidity in epilepsy: basic mechanisms, diagnosis and treatment. McConnell H.W. and Snyder P.J. (eds.) American Psychiatric Press, Washington D.C., pg. 205-244.

McConnell, H. and Duncan, D. *The Use of Antiepileptic Drugs in Psychiatry*. In R. Kerwin (ed): The Maudsley Textbook of Psychiatry (in press).

McElroy, S.L., Keck Jr, P.E., Pope Jr, H.G., *et al.* (1988) Valproate in the treatment of rapid cycling bipolar disorder. *Journal of Clinical Psychopharmacology*, **8**, 275-279.

Pazzagila, P.J., Post, R.M., Ketter, T.A., *et al* (1993). Preliminary controlled trial of nimodipine in ultra-rapid cycling affective dysregulation. *Psychiatry Research*, **49**, 257-272.

Taylor, D., Duncan, D. (1996). Treatment options for rapid-cycling bipolar affective disorder. *Psychiatric Bulletin*, **20**, 601-603.

Taylor, D.M., Duncan, D. (1997). Doses of carbamazepine and valproate in bipolar affective disorder. *Psychiatric Bulletin*, **21**, 221-223.

Treatment of Anxiety

Bazire, S. (1999) *Psychotropic Drug Directory*. Quay Books Division, Dinton, Wilts, U.K.

Group authorship. (1992) Guidelines for the management of patients with generalised anxiety. *Psychiatric Bulletin*, **16**, 560-565.

Lader, M. (1994) Treatment of anxiety. *British Medical Journal*, **309**, 321-324.

Perry, P.J., Alexander, B., Liskow, B.I. (1997) *Psychotropic Drug Handbook, 7th Edition*. American Psychiatric Press, Inc., Washington DC, U.S.A.

Special patient groups

Childhood Psychiatric Illness

Fombonne, E. (1998) *The management of depression in children and adolescents*. In: The Management of Depression. Checkley S. (ed). Blackwell Science Ltd, Washington DC, U.S.A.

Green, W. H. (1995) Child and Adolescent Clinical Psychopharmacology. Williams & Wilkins, Baltimore, U.S.A.

Kumra, S., Frazier, J.A., Jacobsen, L.K. *et al.* (1996). Childhood-onset schizophrenia: a double-blind clozapine-haloperidol comparison. *Archives of General Psychiatry*, **53**, 1090-1097.

McConnell, H. (1985) Catecholamine metabolism in the attention deficit disorder. *Medical Hypotheses* 17(4):305-313.

Taylor, E. (1994) *Physical Treatments*. In: Rutter M., Taylor E. & Hersov L. (eds) Child and Adolescent Psychiatry: Modern Approaches. Third edition. Blackwell Scientific Publications, Oxford, U.K. pg. 880-899.

Weiner, J.M., (ed) (1996) Diagnosis and Psychopharmacology of Childhood and Adolescent Disorders. John Wiley and Sons, New York, NY, U.S.A.

Werry, J.S., Aman, M.G. (1993) Practitioner's Guide to Psychoactive Drugs for Children and Adolescents. Plenum Publishing Corporation, New York, NY, U.S.A.

The Elderly

Breitner, J.C.S., Welsh, K.A. (1995) Diagnosis and management of memory loss and cognitive disorders among elderly persons. *Psychiatric Services*, **46**, 29-35.

Coffey, C.E., Cummings, J.L. (1994). Textbook of geriatric neuropsychiatry. American Psychiatric Press, Inc., Washington D.C. , U.S.A.

Grossberg, G.T., Manepalli, J. (1995) The older patient with psychotic symptoms. *Psychiatric Services*, **46**, 55-54.

Kennedy, G.J. (1995) The geriatric syndrome of late-life depression. *Psychiatric Services,* **46**, 43.

McCall, W.V. (1995) Management of primary sleep disorders among elderly persons. *Psychiatric Services*, **46**, 49-55.

McConnell H., Duffy J. (1994) Neuropsychiatric Effects of Medical Treatment in the Elderly. In Geriatric

Neuropsychiatry (J. Cummins and E. Coffey, Eds), American Psychiatric Press, Washington, D.C., U.S.A.

McConnell, H., Snyder, P.J. (1998) Electroencephalography in the elderly. In P.Nussbaum (Ed.), Handbook of Neuropsychology and Aging. A volume in the *Critical Issues in Neuropsychology* series (E.E. Puente & C.R. Reynolds, Eds.). Plenum Press, New York, USA

Norman, J., Redfern, S.J. (1997) Mental Health Care for Elderly People. Churchill Livingston, New York, U.S.A.

Reynolds, C.F. (1992) Treatment of depression in special populations. *Journal of Clinical Psychiatry,* **53** (Suppl.9), 45.

Schneider, L.S. (1996) Overview of generalized anxiety disorder in the elderly. *Journal of Clincal Psychiatry,* **57** (Suppl 7), 34-45.

Smith, S.L., Sherrill, K.A., Colenda, C.C. (1995) Assessing and treating anxiety in elderly persons. *Psychiatric Services,* **46**, 36-42.

Pregnancy and Lactation

Adis International Ltd. (1995) Neuropsychotherapeutics and breast-feeding – assess the risk: benefit ratio. *Drugs & Therapy Perspectives,* **6**, 10-12.

Adis International Ltd. (1998) Postpartum psychiatric disorders: identify early and treat aggressively. *Drugs & Therapy Perspectives,* **11**, 8-10.

Altshuler, L.L., Cohen, L., Szuba, M.P. *et al.* (1996) Pharmacologic management of psychiatric illness during pregnancy: dilemmas and guidelines. *American Journal of Psychiatry,* **153**, 592-606.

Altshuler, L.L., Hendrick, V.C. (1996) Pregnancy and psychotropic medication: changes in blood levels. *Journal of Clinical Psychopharmacology,* **16**, 78-80.

Altshuler, L.L., Hendrick, V., Cohen, L.S. (1998) Course of mood and anxiety disorders during pregnancy and the postpartum period. *Journal of Clinical Psychiatry,* **59** (suppl 2), 29-33.

Association of the British Pharmaceutical Industry (1998) Compendium of Data Sheets and Summaries of Product Characteristics. Datapharm Publications Ltd., London, U.K.

Bazire, S. (1999) Psychotropic Drug Directory. Quay Books, Salisbury, U.K.

Begg, E.J., Atkinson, H.C., Darlow, B.A. (1996) *Guide to safety of drugs in breast feeding.* In: Avery's Drug Treatment, 4th Edition. Speight, T.M. and Holford, N.H.G. (eds.) Adis International Ltd., Sydney, Australia.

Buist, A. (1997) Postpartum psychiatric disorders: guidelines for management. *CNS Drugs,* **8**, 113-123.

Chisholm, C.A., Kuller, J.A. (1997) A guide to the safety of CNS-active agents during breastfeeding. *Drug Safety,* **17**, 127-142.

Cohen, L.S., Rosenbaum, J.F. (1998) Psychotropic drug use during pregnancy: weighing the risks. *Journal of Clinical Psychiatry,* **59** (suppl 2), 18-28.

Cooper, P.J., Murray, L. (1998) Postnatal depression. *British Medical Journal,* **316**, 1884-1886.

Dolovich, L.S., Addis, A., Vaillancourt, J.M.R., *et al.* (1998) Benzodiazepine use in pregnancy and major malformations or oral cleft: meta-analysis of cohort and case-control studies. *British Medical Journal,* **317**, 829–843.

Duncan, D.A., Taylor, D.M. (1995). Which antidepressants are safe to use in breast-feeding mothers? *Psychiatric Bulletin*, **19**, 551-552.

Dwight, M.M., Walker, E.A. (1998) Depressive disorders during pregnancy and postpartum. *Current Opinion in Psychiatry*, **11**, 85-88.

Goldstein, D.J. (1995) Effects of third trimester fluoxetine exposure on the newborn. *Journal of Clinical Psychopharmacology*, **15**, 417-420.

Kendell, R.E., Chalmers, J.C., Platz, C. (1987) Epidemiology of puerperal psychoses. *British Journal of Psychiatry*, **150** 662-673.

Kulin, N.A., Pastuszak, A., Sage, S.R. *et al.* (1998) Pregnancy outcome following maternal use of the new selective serotonin reuptake inhibitors: a prospective controlled multicenter study. *JAMA,* **279**, 609-610.

Lee, A., Donaldson, S. (1995). Drugs In Pregnancy – Psychiatric and neurological disorders: part 1. *The Pharmaceutical Journal*, **254**, 87-90.

Llewellyn, A., Stowe, Z.N. (1998) Psychotropic medications in lactation. *Journal of Clinical Psychiatry*, **59** (suppl 2), 41-52.

Llewellyn, A.M., Stowe, Z.N., Nemeroff, C.B. (1997) Depression during pregnancy and the puerperium. *Journal of Clincal Psychiatry*, **58** (suppl 15), 26-32.

Loebstein, R., Koren, G. (1997) Pregnancy outcome and neurodevelopment of children exposed in utero to psychoactive drugs: the Motherisk Experience. *Journal of Psychiatry and Neurosciences*, **22**, 192-197.

Marks, M., Kumar, R.C. (1998) *Depression after childbirth.* In: The Management of Depression. Checkley, S. (ed). Blackwell Science Ltd., Oxford, U.K.

McElhatton, P.R. (1992) The use of phenothiazines during pregnancy and lactation. *Reproductive Toxicology*, **6**, 474-490.

McElhatton, P.R. (1994) A review of the effects of benzodiazepine use during pregnancy and lactation. *Reproductive Toxicology*, **8**, 461-475.

McElhatton, P.R., Garbis, H.M., Elefant, E. *et al.* (1996) The outcome of pregnancy in 689 women exposed to therapeutics doses of antidepressants. *Reproductive Toxicology*, **10**, 285-294.

Murray, L., Cooper, P.J. (1997) Postpartum depression and child development. *Psychological Medicine*, **27**, 253-260.

Nonacs, R., Cohen, L.S. (1998) Postpartum mood disorders: diagnosis and treatment guidelines. *Journal of Clinical Psychiatry*, **59** (suppl 2), 34-40.

Nulman, I., Rovet, J., Stewart, D.E. *et al.* (1997) Neurodevelopment of children exposed in utero to antidepressant drugs. *The New England Journal of Medicine*, **336**, 258-262.

Spigset, O., Hägg, S. (1998) Excretion of psychotropic drugs into breast milk: pharmacokinetic overview and therapeutic implications. *CNS Drugs*, **9**, 111-134

Trixler, M., Tenyi, T. (1997) Antipsychotic use in pregnancy. *Drug Safety Concepts*, **16**, 403-410.

Weinberg, M.K., Tronick, E.Z. (1998) The impact of maternal psychiatric illness on infant development. *Journal of Clinical Psychiatry*, **59** (suppl 2), 53-61.

Yonkers, K.A., Little, B.B., March, D. (1998) Lithium during pregnancy: drug effects and their therapeutic implications. *CNS Drugs*, **9**, 261-269.

Yoshida, K., Kumar, R. (1996) Breast feeding and psychotropic drugs. *International Review of Psychiatry*, **8**, 117-124.

Yoshida, K., Smith, B., Kumar, R. (1999) Psychotropic drugs in mothers' milk: a comprehensive review of assay methods, pharmacokinetics and of safety of breast-feeding. *Journal of Psychopharmacology*, **13**, 76-92.

Medical Co-Morbidity

Hale, A.S. (1993) New antidepressants: use in high-risk patients. *Journal of Clinical Psychiatry*, **54** (Suppl. 8), 61-70.

Haynal, A., Pasini, W. (1984) Medicine Psychosomatique. Masson, Paris, France.

Masand, P.S., Tesar, G.E. (1996) Use of stimulants in the medically ill. *The Psychiatric Clinics of North America*, **19**, 515-547.

Patten, S.B. and Love, E.J. (1994) Neuropsychiatric adverse drug reactions: passive reports to health and welfare. Canada's adverse drug reaction database (1965-present). *International Journal of Psychiatry in Medicine*, **24**, 45-62.

Reynolds, C.F. (1992) Treatment of depression in special populations. *Journal of Clinical Psychiatry*, **53** (Suppl. 9), 45-53.

Stoudemire, A. (1996) New antidepressant drugs and the treatment of depression in the medically ill patient. *The Psychiatric Clinics of North America*, **19**, 495-514

Hepatic impairment

Daly, M.J. Choice of neuroleptic in liver disease. *St James's Drug Information Centre* (letter 1999).

Daly, M.J. Choice of antidepressant in liver disease. *St James's Drug Information Centre* (letter 1998).

Davis, M., (1991). Hepatotoxicity of antidepressants. *International Clinical Psychopharmacology*, **6**, 97-103.

Finlayson, N.D.C. (1994) Drugs and the liver. *Medicine International*, 455-459.

Morgan, D.J., McLean, A.J. (1995). Clinical pharmacokinetic and pharmacodynamic considerations in patients with liver disease. *Clinical Pharmacokinetics*, **29**, 370-391.

Wanke, L.A., Silbernagel, R. L. (1999) Drug Consults: Antidepressant use in chronic liver disease. *Micromedex Inc.*, **99**, 1-5

Renal Impairment

Bennett, W.M., Aronoff, G.R., Golper, T.A. *et al.* (1991) *Drug prescribing in renal failure*. 2nd Ed. American College of Physicians, Philadelphia, U.S.A.

Bergstrom, R.F., Beasley Jr., C.M., Levy, N.B., *et al.* (1993) The effects of renal and hepatic disease on the pharmacokinetics, renal tolerance, and risk-benefit profile of fluoxetine. *International Clinical Psychopharmacology*, **8**, 261-266.

Doyle, G.D., Laher, M., Kelly, J.G. *et al.* (1989**)** The pharmacokinetics of paroxetine in renal impairment. *Acta Psychiatrica. Scandinavica*, **80**, 89-90.

Schrier, R.W., Gambertoglio, J.G., (eds) (1991). *Handbook of drug therapy in liver and kidney disease*. Little, Brown and Co., Boston, U.S.A.

Snoeck, E., Van Peer, A., Sack, M. *et al*. (1995) Influence of age, renal and liver impairment on the pharmacokinetics of risperidone in man. *Psychopharmacology* **122**, 223-229.

Psychiatric Effects of Medical therapies

Brown T.M., Stoudemire A. (1998) Psychiatric side effects of prescription and over-the-counter medicines. American Psychiatric Press Inc. Washington DC, USA.

McConnell H., Duffy J. (1994) Neuropsychiatric Effects of Medical Treatment in the Elderly. In Geriatric Neuropsychiatry (J. Cummins and E. Coffey, Eds), American Psychiatric Press, Washington, D.C., U.S.A.

Saravay, S.M. (1996) Psychiatric interventions in the medically ill: outcome and effectiveness research. *Psychiatric Clinics of North America*. **19**, 467-480.

Stoudemire, A. (1996) New antidepressant drugs and the treatment of depression in the medically ill patient. . *Psychiatric Clinics of North America* **19**, 495-513.

Neuropsychiatry

Aimard G., Vighetto A., Bret Ph., *et al*. (1989) Theraputique Neuropsychiatrique. Masson, Paris

Fogel, B.S., Schiffer, R.B (eds) (1996) Neuropsychiatry. Williams & Wilkins, Baltimore, U.S.A.

Lishman, A. (1998) Organic Psychiatry, Third Edition. Blackwell Science, Oxford, U.K.

McConnell H.W. and Snyder P.J. (1998) Psychiatric Co-morbidity in epilepsy: basic mechanisms, diagnosis and treatment. American Psychiatric Press, Washington DC, U.S.A.

Ruta, D.A. (1997) Neurology and guideline development. *Neurology*, **1**, 1-4.

Yudofsky, S.C. and Hales, R.E. (eds) (1997) American Psychiatric Press Textbook of Neuropsychiatry. AP Press, Washington DC, USA

Alcohol and Substance Misuse

Duncan, D., Taylor, D. (1996). Chlormethiazole or chlordiazepoxide in alcohol detoxification. *Psychiatric Bulletin*, **20**, 599-601.

Ling, W., Compton, P., Rawson, R. *et al*. (1996) Neuropsychiatry of Alcohol and Drug Abuse. In Fogel, B.S., Schiffer, R.B (eds) Neuropsychiatry. Williams & Wilkins, Baltimore, U.S.A. Pg. 679-722.

Alzheimer's Disease and Dementia

Alexopoulos, G.S. (1996) The treatment of depressed demented patients. *Journal of Clinical Psychiatry*, **57** (Suppl. 14), 14-20.

Anon. (1998) Donepezil Update. *Drug and Therapeutics Bulletin*, **36**, 60-61.

Corey-Bloom, J., Anand, R., Veach, J. (1998) A randomized trial evaluating the efficacy and safety of ENA 713 (rivastigmine tartrate), a new acetylcholinesterase inhibitor, in patients with mild to moderately severe Alzheimer's disease. *International Journal of Geriatric Psychopharmacology,* **1**, 55-65.

Lott, A.D., McElroy, S.L., Keys, M.A. (1995) Valproate in the treatment of behavioral agitation in elderly patients with dementia. *The Journal of Neuropsychiatry and Clinical Neurosciences,* **7**, 314-319.

Lyketsos, C.G., Corazzini, K., Steele, C.D. (1996) Guidelines for the use of tacrine in Alzheimer's disease: clinical application and effectiveness. *Journal of Neuropsychiatry,* **8**, 67-73.

Noble, S., Wagstaff, A.J. (1997) Propentofylline. *CNS Drugs,* **8**, 257-264.

Rabins, P.V. (1996) Developing treatment guidelines for Alzheimer's disease and other dementias. *Journal of Clinical Psychiatry,* **57** (Suppl. 14), 37-38.

Rogers, S.L., Doody, R.S., Mohs, R.C. (1998) Donepezil improves cognition and global function in Alzheimer Disease: a 15-week, double-blind, placebo-controlled study. *Archives of Internal Medicine,* **158**, 1021-1031.

Rogers, S.L., Farlow, M.R., Doody, R.S. *et al.* (1998) A 24-week, double-blind, placebo-controlled trial of donepezil in patients with Alzheimer's disease. *Neurology,* **50**, 136-145.

Rogers, S., Friedhoff, L. (1998) Long-term efficacy and safety of donepezil in the treatment of Alzheimer's disease: an interim analysis of the results of a US multicentre open label extension study. *European Neuropsychopharmacology,* **8**, 67-75.

Schneider, L.S. (1996) New therapeutic approaches to Alzheimer's disease. *Journal of Clinical Psychiatry,* **57** **(Suppl. 14)**, 30-36.

Standing Medical Advisory Committee (1998) The use of donepezil for Alzheimer's disease. *Department of Health, U.K.,* 1-3.

Tariot, P.N. (1996) Treatment strategies for agitation and psychosis in dementia. *Journal of Clinical Psychiatry,* **57** (Suppl. 14), 21-29.

Zayas, E.M., Grossberg, G.T. (1996) Treating the agitated Alzheimer patient. *Journal of Clinical Psychiatry,* **57** (Suppl. 7), 46-51.

Epilepsy

Appleton, R.E. (1998) Guideline may help in prescribing vigabatrin. *British Medical Journal,* **317**, 1322.

Betts, T. (1998) *Epilepsy, Psychiatry and Learning Difficulty.* Martin Dunitz, London, U.K.

Brown, S., Betts, T., Chadwick, D., *et al.* (1993) An Epilepsy Needs Document. *Seizure,* **2**, 91-103.

Epilepsy Task Force. *Medical Treatment Guidelines.* Epilepsy Task Force/Joint Epilepsy Council, 1994

Fenwick, P.B.C. (1988) Seizures, EEG discharges and Behaviour. In Epilepsy, Behaviour and Cognitive Function. MR Trimble and EH Reynolds (eds) John Wiley and Sons, Chichester, U.K., 51-66.

McConnell, H.W., Duncan, D. (1998a) *Behavioural effects of antiepileptic drugs.* In: Psychiatric co-morbidity in epilepsy: basic mechanisms, diagnosis and treatment. McConnell H.W. and Snyder P.J. (eds.) American Psychiatric Press, Washington D.C., U.S.A., 205-244.

McConnell, H.W., Duncan D. (1998b) *The Treatment of Psychiatric Co-Morbidity in Epilepsy.* In: Psychiatric Co-morbidity in epilepsy: basic mechanisms, diagnosis and treatment. McConnell H.W. and Snyder P.J. (eds) Washington DC, American Psychiatric Press, U.S.A. Pg. 245-361.

McConnell, H., Duncan, D., Taylor, D. (1997) Choice of neuroleptics in epilepsy. *Psychiatric Bulletin,* **21**, 642-645.

McConnell, H., Duncan, D. The Use of Antiepileptic Drugs in psychiatry. In: R. Kerwin (ed): The Maudsley Textbook of Psychiatry (in press).

McConnell, H., Duncan, D. Psychiatric Co-Morbidity in Epilepsy. In: R. Kerwin (ed): The Maudsley Textbook of Psychiatry (in press).

McConnell, H. Snyder, P.J. (1998) Electroencephalography in the elderly. In: P.Nussbaum (Ed.), Handbook of Neuropsychology and Aging. A volume in the *Critical Issues in Neuropsychology* series (E.E. Puente & C.R. Reynolds, Eds.). Plenum Press, New York, USA.

McConnell H.W., Snyder P.J. (1998) Psychiatric Co-morbidity in epilepsy: basic mechanisms, diagnosis and treatment. American Psychiatric Press, Washington DC, U.S.A.

McConnell H.W., Snyder P.J. The Clinicians's Perspective of Quality of Life in Epilepsy. In: Quality of Life in Epilepsy, G. Baker and A. Jacoby (eds), in press.

O'Connor, R., Cox,. J., Couglan, M. (1996) *Diagnosis and Management of Epilepsy in General Practice.* Irish College of General Practitioners, Dublin.

Report of Quality Standards Subcommittee of the American Academy of Neurology. (1998) Practice parameter: management issues for women with epilepsy (summary statement). *Neurology,* **51**, 944-947.

Scottish Intercollegiate Guideline Network (SIGN) (1997) *Diagnosis and Management of Adult Epilepsy in Primary and Secondary Care,* SIGN, Edinburgh

Shorvon, S. (ed) (1996) The Treatment of Epilepsy. Blackwell Scientific, Oxford, U.K.

Snyder, P.J., McConnell, H. (1998) Epilepsy in the Elderly. In: P. Nussbaum (Ed.) Handbook of Neuro-psychology and Aging. A volume in the Critical Issues in Neuropsychology series (A.E. Puente & C.R. Reynolds, Eds.). Plenum Press, New York, U.S.A.

Tomson, T., Gram, L., Sillanpaa, M. *et al* (eds.) (1997) Epilepsy and Pregnancy. Rightson Medical Publishing, Petersfield, UK.

Trimble, M.R., Ring, H., Schmitz, B. (1996) Neuropsychiatric Aspects of Epilepsy. In: Fogel, B.S., Schiffer, R.B (eds) Neuropsychiatry. Williams & Wilkins, Baltimore. U.S.A.

Wallace, H., Shorvon, S., Hopkins, A., *et al.* (1997) Adults with Poorly Controlled Epilepsy, Part I. Clinical Guidelines for Treatment, Royal College of Physicians of London,.

Wilder, B.J. (1998) Management of Epilepsy: Consensus Conference on Current Clinical Practice, *Neurology,* **51 (5)** Suppl. 4.

Gilles de la Tourette's Syndrome

Chase, T.N., Friedhoff, A.J., Cohen, D.J. Tourette syndrome genetics, neurobiology and treatment. *Advances in Neurology* (1992) **Vol.58** Raven Press, New York

Comings, D.E. (1990) Tourette's Syndrome and Human Behavior. Hope Press, Duarte, CA, U.S.A.

Peterson, B.S. (1996) Considerations of natural history and pathophysiology in the psychopharmacology of Tourette's Syndrome. *Journal of Clinical Psychiatry,* **57**,24-34.

Robertson, M. (1996) Gilles de la Tourette Syndrome and Obsessive-Compulsive Disorder. In: Fogel, B.S., Schiffer, R.B (eds) Neuropsychiatry. Williams & Wilkins, Baltimore. Pg. 827-870.

Sandor, P. (1995) Clinical management of Tourette's syndrome and associated disorders. *Canadian Journal of Psychiatry,* **40**, 577-583.

Head Injury

Barrett, K. (1991) Treating organic abulia with bromocriptine and lisuride. *Journal of Neurology, Neurosurgery and Psychiatry,* **54**, 718-721.

Brooke, M.M., Patterson, D.R., Questad, K.A. *et al.* (1992) The treatment of agitation during initial hospitalisation after traumatic brain injury. *Archives of Physical Medicine and Rehabilitation*, **73**, 917-921.

Feeney, D.M., Gonzalez, A., Law, W.A. (1982) Amphetamine, haloperidol and experience interact to affect rate of recovery after motor cortex injury. *Science*, **217**, 855-857.

Geracioti, T.D. (1994) Valproic acid treatment of episodic explosiveness related to brain injury. *Journal of Clinical Psychiatry, **55**,* 416-417.

Greendyke, R.M., Kanter, D.R. (1986) Therapeutic effects of pindolol on behavioural disturbances associated with organic brain disease: A double-blind study. *Journal of Clinical Psychiatry*, **47**, 423-426.

Lewin, J., Sumners, D. (1992) Successful treatment of episodic dyscontrol with carbamazepine. *British Journal of Psychiatry,* **161**, 261-262.

Lishman, W.A. (1998) Organic Psychiatry, Third Edition. Blackwell Science: London, U.K.

McConnell, H.W., Duncan D. (1998b) *The Treatment of Psychiatric Co-Morbidity in Epilepsy.* In: Psychiatric Co-morbidity in epilepsy: basic mechanisms, diagnosis and treatment. McConnell H.W. and Snyder P.J. (eds), Washington DC, American Psychiatric Press, U.S.A. Pg. 245-361.

Pourcher, E., Filteau,M.J., Bouchard, R.H., *et al.* (1994) Efficacy of the combination of buspirone and carbamazepine in early posttraumatic delirium. *American Journal of Psychiatry*, **151**, 150-151.

Robinson, R.G., Jorge, R. (1994) Mood Disorders, in *Neuropsychiatry of Traumatic Brain Injury*, (Eds) J.M. Silver, S.C. Yudofsky and R.E. Hale. American Psychiatry Press Inc: Washington, U.S.A.

Multiple Sclerosis

Mahler, M.E. (1992) Behavioral manifestations associated with Multiple Sclerosis. *Psychiatric Clinics of North America*, **15**, 427-437.

Scott, T.F., Allen, D., Price, T.R.P. *et al.* (1996) Characterization of major depression symptoms in Multiple Sclerosis patients. *Journal of Neuropsychiatry and Clinical Neurosciences* **8**, 318-323.

Scott, T., Nussbaum, P., McConnell, H. *et al.* (1996) Measurement of Treatment Response to Sertraline in Depressed Multiple Sclerosis Patients Using The Carroll Scale. *Neurology Research,* **7,** 421-422,

Parkinson's Disease

Cole, S.A., Woodard, J.L., Juncos, J.L., *et al.* (1996) Depression and disability in Parkinson's Disease. *Journal of Neuropsychiatry and Clinical Neurosciences,* **8**, 20-25.

Factor, S.A., Molho, E.S., Brown, D.L. (1995) Combined clozapine and electroconvulsive therapy for the treatment of drug-induced psychosis in Parkinson's disease. *The Journal of Neuropsychiatry and Clinical Neurosciences*, **7**, 304-307.

Hegeman-Richard, I., Schiffer, R.B., Kurlan, R. (1996) Anxiety and Parkinson's Disease. *Journal of Neuropsychiatry and Clinical Neurosciences*, **8**, 383-392.

Klaassen, T., Verhey, F.R.J., Sneijders, G.H.J.M. *et al.* (1995) Treatment of depression in Parkinson's Disease: a meta-analysis. *Journal of Neuropsychiatry and Clinical Neurosciences* **7**, 281-286.

Mendis, T., Barclay, C.L., Mohr, E. (1996) Drug-induced psychosis in Parkinson's Disease: a review of management. *CNS Drugs*, **5**, 166-174.

Musser, W.S., Akil, M. (1996) Clozapine as a treatment for psychosis in Parkinson' Disease: A review. *Journal of Neuropsychiatry and Clinical Neurosciences,* **8**, 1-9.

Parsa, M.A. and Bastani, B. (1998) Quetiapine (Seroquel) in the treatment of psychosis in patients with Parkinson's disease. *Journal of Neuropsychiatry and Clinical Neurosciences*, **10**, 216-219.

Pfeiffer, C., Wagner, M.L. (1994) Clozapine therapy for Parkinson's disease and other movement disorders. *American Journal of Hospital Pharmacy*, **51**, 3047-3053.

Wagner, M.L., Defilippi, J.L., Menza, M.A. *et al.* (1996) Clozapine for the treatment of psychosis in Parkinson's Disease: chart review of 49 patients. *Journal of Neuropsychiatry*, **8**, 276-280.

Wolters, E.Ch., Jansen, E.N.H., Tuynman-Qua, H.G., *et al.* (1996) Olanzapine in the treatment of dopaminomimetic psychosis in patients with Parkinson's Disease. *Neurology*, **47**, 1085-1087.

Porphyria

Crimlisk, H.L. (1997). The little imitator B porphyria: a neuropsychiatric disorder. *Journal of Neurology, Neurosurgery, and Psychiatry*, **62**, 319-328.

Lishman, WA (1998) Organic Psychiatry Third Edition, Blackwell Science, Oxford, pp. 567-569.

Stroke

Absher, J.R., Toole, J.F. (1996) Neurobehavioral features of cerebrovascular disease. In: Fogel, B.S., Schiffer, R.B (eds) Neuropsychiatry. Williams & Wilkins, Baltimore, Pg 895-912.

Duncan, D., Sayal, K., McConnell, H. *et al* (1998) Antidepressant interactions with warfarin. *International Clinical Psychopharmacology*, **13**, 87-94.

Graff-Radford, N.R., Biller, J. (1992) Behavioral neurology and stroke. *Psychiatric Clinics of North America*, **15**, 415-425.

Greenblatt D.J., von Moltke L.L., Harmatz, J.S. *et al.* (1998) Drug interactions with newer antidepressants: role of human cytochromes P450. *Journal of Clinical Psychiatry*, **59**(Suppl 15), 19–27.

House, A. (1996) Depression associated with stroke. *Journal of Neuropsychiatry and Clinical Neurosciences*, **8**, 454-457.

Treatment of Medical / Psychiatric Emergencies

Dubin, W.R. (1988). Rapid tranquillisation: antipsychotics of benzodiazepines. *Journal of Clinical Psychiatry*, **49** [suppl. 12], 5-11.

Kerr, I.B., Taylor, D. (1997) Acute disturbed or violent behaviour: principles of treatment. *Journal of Psychopharmacology*, **11**, 271-277.

Pilowsky, L.S., Ring, H., Shine, P.J., *et al.* (1992). Rapid tranquillisation. A survey of emergency prescribing in a general psychiatric hospital. *British Journal of Psychiatry*, **160**, 831-835.

Resnick, M., Burton, B.T. (1984). Droperidol vs haloperidol in the initial management of acutely agitated patients. *Journal of Clinical Psychiatry*, **45**, 298-299.

Adverse Effects of Psychotropic Drugs

Management of Weight Change from Psychotropics

Ackerman, S., Nolan, L.J. (1998) Bodyweight gain induced by psychotropic agents: incidence, mechanisms and management. *CNS Drugs,* **9**, 135-151

Isojärvi, J.I.T., Laatikainen, T.J., Knip, M. *et al.* (1996) Obesity and endocrine disorders in women taking valproate for epilepsy. *Annals of Neurology*, **39**, 579-584.

Pijl, H., Meinders, A.E. (1998) Bodyweight Change as an Adverse Effect of Drug Treatment. *Drug Safety,* **14**, 329-342.

Silverstone T. Body weight changes during treatment with psychotropic drugs (Psychiatrists Information Service Monograph Series No. 1). Janssen Pharmaceuticals, Oxford, UK

Clozapine: Management of adverse effects

Fritze, J., Tilmann, E. (1995). Pirenzepine for clozapine-induced hypersalivation. *Lancet*, **346**, 1034.

Pacia, S.V., Devinsky, O. (1994). Clozapine-related seizures: experience with 5,629 patients. *Neurology*, **44**, 2247-2249.

Taylor, D., Reveley, A., Faivre, F. (1995). Clozapine-induced hypotension treated with moclobemide and Bovril. *British Journal of Psychiatry*, **167**, 409-410.

Antipsychotic – induced akathisia

Adler, L., Angrist, B., Peselow, E. *et al* (1986). A controlled assessment of propranolol in the treatment of neuroleptic-induced akathisia. *British Journal of Psychiatry*, **149**, 42-45.

Fleischhacker, W. W. , Roth, S. D., Kane, J. M. (1990). The pharmacologic treatment of neuroleptic-induced akathisia. *Journal of Clinical Psychopharmacology*, **10**, 12-21.

Weiss, D., Aizenberg, D., Hermesh, H. *et al* (1995). Cyproheptadine treatment of neuroleptic-induced akathisia. *British Journal of Psychiatry*, **167**, 483-486.

Antipsychotic induced hyperprolactinaemia

Duncan, D., Taylor, D. (1995). Treatment of psychotropic-induced hyperprolactinaemia. *Psychiatric Bulletin*, **19**, 755-757.

Neuroleptic Malignant Syndrome

Dent, J. (1996) Diagnosing neuroleptic malignant syndrome. *Psychiatry in Practice*, **Autumn**, 5-8.

Isojärvi, J.I.T., Laatikainen, T.J., Knip, M. *et al.* (1996) Obesity and endocrine disorders in women taking valproate for epilepsy. *Annals of Neurology*, **39**, 579-584

Koponen, H., Repo, E., Lepola, U. (1991) Long-term outcome after neuroleptic malignant syndrome. *Acta Psychiatrica Scandinavica*, **84**, 550-551.

Levenson, J.L. (1985) Neuroleptic malignant syndrome. *American Journal of Psychiatry*, **142**, 1137-1145.

Lɪ.ʰman, W.A. (1998) Organic Psychiatry, Third Edition. Blackwell Science, London, U.K.

Modestin, J., Toffler, G., Drescher, J.P. (1992) Neuroleptic malignant syndrome: results of a prospective study. *Psychiatry Research*, **44**, 251-256.

Spivak, B., Gonen, N., Mester, R., *et al.* (1996) Neuroleptic malignant syndrome associated with abrupt withdrawal of anticholinergic agents. *International Clinical Psychopharmacology*, **11**, 207-209.

Wells, A.J., Sommi, R.W., Crismon, M.L. (1988) Neuroleptic rechallenge after neuroleptic malignant syndrome: case report and literature review. *Drug Intelligence and Clincial Pharmacy*, **22**, 475-480.

Tardive Dyskinesia

Duncan, D., McConnell, H., Taylor, D. (1997) Tardive dyskinesia – how is it prevented and treated? *Psychiatric Bulletin*, **21**, 422-425.

Joseph, A.B., Young, R.R. (1992) Movement disorders in neurology and neuropsychiatry. Blackwell Scientific Publications, Oxford, U.K.

Keghavan, M.S., Kennedy, J.S. (1992) *Drug induced dysfunction in psychiatry.* Hemisphere Publishing, New York, NY, U.S.A.

Appendices

Appendix I

Antibiotic Use in Psychiatry

General Guidelines

❖ Suitable samples of infected material should be sent for microbiological examination before initiating empirical antimicrobial therapy. Contact Microbiology for advice about sampling and therapy.

❖ BNF doses should be followed.

❖ When appropriate, oral therapy should be instituted. Prescriptions should be for a 5 day course and then reviewed. However, in the case of chronic diseases which require long term therapy, e.g. osteomyelitis, neurosyphilis or tuberculosis, advice should be sought from the Infection Control Team or other appropriate specialists.

❖ If after 48 hours' therapy clinical improvement is not observed, or treatment shown to be inappropriate, Microbiology should be consulted.

❖ [i] Intravenous/intramuscular antibiotics are not listed and will usually not be reported as many Psychiatric nursing staff are not qualified to administer them. However where these routes are considered essential, please contact Microbiology, Pharmacy, or other appropriate specialists.

[ii] The circumstances in which the parenteral route should be considered are if:

a] the patient is seriously ill,

b] the infection is sensitive to a parenteral-only agent,

c] the infection has not responded to an appropriate course of oral therapy,

d] the patient is unable to take medication orally.

❖ Topical antibiotics, including mupirocin should be avoided unless recommended by the Infection Control Team or other appropriate specialists.

❖ Where the oral route is contraindicated, metronidazole can be administered rectally. Please contact Microbiology or Pharmacy.

❖ Infected samples of urine from patients who are catheterised should not lead to automatic treatment unless systemic infection is present. Consult Microbiology.

❖ Products to which the patients are known to be allergic should NEVER be administered. NB. Allergy to penicillins is rarely associated with cross sensitivity to cephalosporins. If in doubt contact Microbology or Pharmacy.

Recommended Treatment of Common Infections

For Urinary Tract Infections [UTI]:

1st line: trimethoprim, amoxycillin or cefadroxil.
2nd line: nalidixic acid or co-amoxiclav.
Multiple resistant organisms: ciprofloxacin.

For Respiratory Tract Infections:

1st line: amoxycillin or erythromycin. If not improving in 24 hours, consult Microbiology.
2nd line: clarithromycin [3 day course] or co-amoxiclav.

For fungal infections:

Nystatin suspension for oral infections; clotrimazole for skin infections;
fluconazole for systemic or resistant skin infections.
Terbinafine may be used in some instances. Consult Microbiology.

For throat infections - Streps:

Penicillin, erythromycin or amoxycillin.

For wounds / ulcers and pressure sores - topical antibiotics may not be used. In most
cases wound irrigation and cleaning are sufficient. If there are clinical signs and symptoms of cellulitis consult Microbiology.

For Pelvic Inflammatory Disease and vaginal discharge

Collect high vaginal swab. If Neisseria gonorrhoeae [the gonococcus, GC] is excluded, treat:
1st line: metronidazole [400mg bd for 5-7 days] PLUS doxycycline [100mg bd for 14 days].
Erythromycin may be substituted for doxycycline if doxycycline is not tolerated [500mg qds for 14 days].
For GC consult Microbiology.

For gastroenteritis

Antibiotics are not generally indicated. The Infection Control Team or other appropriate specialist must be informed and faecal samples must be sent to the laboratory.

For eyes and ears - topical

For advice, particularly if otitis media is suspected, consult Microbiology or Pathology.
Eyes - 1st line: chloramphenicol drops/ointment
Ears - 1st line: chloramphenicol drops. [2nd line: neomycin, polymyxin]

For tuberculosis

A chest physician must be consulted for recommendations. Tuberculosis is a notifiable disease and the Infection Control Team must be alerted immediately if the disease is suspected.

Treatment of Specific Organisms

For Staph aureus:

Flucloxacillin, or sodium fusidate PLUS erythromycin.

For MRSA:

Contact the Infection Control Team or other appropriate specialist and see the MRSA policy in the current Infection Control Policy for suitable topical preparations and protocols for treatment of colonisation and infection.

For Anaerobes:

Metronidazole.

First Line Agents

Antibiotic	Form	Strength	Usual dose
AMOXYCILLIN	capsules	250mg	250-500mg tds
	suspension	250mg/5ml	
CEFADROXIL	capsules	500mg	500mg bd
	suspension	500mg /5ml	
DOXYCYCLINE	capsules	100mg	200mg stat, 100mg od
ERYTHROMYCIN	tablets	250mg	250-500mg qds/tds
FLUCLOXACILLIN	capsules	250mg	250-500mg qds
METRONIDAZOLE	tablets	200mg	200-400mg tds
	suppositories	1g	1g tds x 3/7 then bd
TRIMETHOPRIM	tablets	200mg	200mg bd

Antifungal	form	strength	usual dose
* Nystatin	mouthwash	100,000 units/ml	1ml qds
Fluconazole	capsules	50mg	50mg od
Clotrimazole	pessaries	500mg	one stat.

[* topical effect only: not absorbed systemically]

Second Line Agents

Recommended by Microbiology in the case of resistant organisms

Antibiotic	form	strength	usual dose
CIPROFLOXACIN	tablets	250mg	250mg bd
CO-AMOXICLAV	tablets	375mg	1 tds
NALIDIXIC ACID	tablet	500mg	1g qds
SODIUM FUSIDATE	tablets	250mg	500mg tds
TEICOPLANIN	injection	200mg	400mg stat, 200mg/d

Note:

These guidelines were developed specifically for the Bethlem and Maudsley NHS Trust and may be different in many respects from policies in other hospitals. Always consult Microbiology, Pathology or Pharmacy departments if in any doubt about antibiotic prescribing. At the Maudsley, contact numbers are:

Microbiology	*2189*
Pharmacy	*2317*
Infection Control	*2189*
Pathology	*2189*

Appendix II

Notes on Guidelines

These guidelines are based on a variety of types of evidence to form this systematically developed statement to assist clinicians in deciding about appropriate care for individual patients in specific circumstances. It represents an act of dedication on behalf of the Authors / Editors who have compiled it, sharing a vision of such efforts improving the prescribing of psychotropics and the lives of the patients. It recognises the problems inherent in large committees producing guidelines, which sometimes have only a vague relation to actual clinical problems encountered by doctors and pharmacists on a daily basis. These guidelines differ then from a 'standard of care' developed by such a committee and based exclusively on evidence-based practice.

The Authors / Editors have produced this volume in its entirety and, in the process, have sought the consultation of various consultants at the Maudsley and Bethlem Hospitals, the Institute of Psychiatry, and international experts from the world over. It is primarily thus a 'consultation document' based on expertise in many aspects of psychiatry for which there are insufficient data to form a standard of care around large well-controlled trials. The Authors / Editors have collected the data for this publication from the following types of evidence: (1) systematic review of randomised controlled trials, (2) review of well-designed controlled trials without randomisation, (3) evidence from well-designed quasi-experimental research, (4) evidence from descriptive studies and case-controlled studies, (5) evidence from expert committees, or world-recognised experts in various aspects of Psychiatry, (6) systematic review of case reports, and (7) a critical analysis of "hypothesis-driven prescribing".

The Authors / Editors have accumulated the above evidence in three phases. In the first instance this has meant an extensive review of the literature, including countless Medline searches, other online database searches, reviews of personal and public libraries and of published and unpublished data. It has also included many web searches and systematic reviews of others' Guidelines from other hospitals in the UK, other countries and international professional organisations. In the second phase of the development of this project, there was extensive consultation from individuals known to have particular expertise in specific areas of Psychiatry. This has included experts from the UK, North America, Australia, New Zealand, the Middle East and Europe. This was achieved in ward round settings, by mail, email and through the use of an International Consensus Conference with videoconferencing. This Consensus Conference was organised by TEAM – Towards Education for All with Multimedia – a non-profit organisation dedicated to the provision of a global network for medical education (102226.74@compuserve.com). This represents a unique approach to Guideline development by an independent non-profit organisation. It also involved both open and closed peer review from publication of many of the ideas presented here in the Drug Information Quarterly, the Psychiatric Bulletin and other professional journals. The third phase of the project involved collating the diverse opinions and coming to agreed consensus amongst the Authors / Editors as to which information represents the most reliable and sensible approach to every day clinical problems. Many of the problems addressed here started as queries from the National Drug Information service. The collation of the above evidence was finally edited into this volume.

These Guidelines then do not represent a view of the typical local practice on Denmark Hill. Nor do they represent a document prepared by a committee reflecting meta-analyses of randomised controlled trials. For many of the questions posed to the National Drug Information Service which have filtered into this document do not have such ready answers. The day-to-day clinical situations of the Psychiatric Pharmacist and Psychiatrist often are not answerable (except by hypothesis-driven enquiry) from the paucity of data available.

These guidelines – now in their fifth edition – represent a constantly changing field. In our process to improve, we value open peer commentary and welcome suggestions for future editions. The effectiveness of guidelines in improving the quality of patient care is well documented. These Guidelines have become an institution in the UK. We now welcome their internationalisation and, with it, a broader scope of both evidence-driven and hypothesis-driven enquiry to remind us how far we have to go in our striving to improve the quality of life and mental health of our patients.